Anti Inflammatory Diet Cookbook For Beginners 2024

The Complete Guide to Quick and Easy Delicious Recipes to Help Reduce Inflammation, Boost Your Immune System And Improve Optimal Health.

Bonus: 28 Day Meal Plan for Anti Inflammatory Diet.

ANNE .J. BAKER

Anne .J. Baker

COPYRIGHT

Copyright © Anne .J. Baker, 2024

All rights reserved. No part of this publication may be reproduced, distributed, or transmitted in any form or by any means, including photocopying, recording, or other electronic or mechanical methods, without the prior written permission of the publisher, except in the case of brief quotations embodied in critical reviews and certain other noncommercial uses permitted by copyright law.

DISCLAIMER

The content in this book is solely for educational and informational purposes and should not be considered as medical advice. This content is not meant to replace professional medical advice, diagnosis, or treatment. Always consult a qualified health provider for any queries about a medical problem.

The book's recipes and nutritional suggestions are founded on fundamental concepts of nutrition and the anti-inflammatory diet. Although attempts have been made to guarantee precision and thoroughness, individual dietary requirements and tastes may differ. Prior to making substantial alterations to your diet, it is crucial to get guidance from a trained dietitian or nutritionist, particularly if you have any current health conditions or concerns.

TABLE OF CONTENTS

INTRODUCTION

Welcome to the Anti-Inflammatory Diet Cookbook for Beginners! I'm Anne J. Baker, a passionate nutritionist dedicated to helping individuals enhance their health and vitality through the power of food. Over the years, I've had the opportunity to mentor folks on their journey to increased well-being, and I've experienced firsthand the remarkable impact that modest dietary adjustments can have on general health.

In today's fast-paced world, many of us are continually assaulted with processed foods, sugary drinks, and unhealthy convenience options. As a result, chronic inflammation has become a prevalent issue, contributing to a range of health problems, including heart disease, arthritis, diabetes, and more. But here's the good news: We have the potential to counteract inflammation and restore our health by making deliberate choices about what we consume.

The Anti-Inflammatory Diet Cookbook for Beginners is your thorough guide to embracing a nourishing way of eating that not only tastes wonderful but also helps your body's natural healing processes. Whether you're brand new to the concept of anti-inflammatory eating or seeking fresh inspiration to rejuvenate your meals, this book is meant to meet you where you are on your health journey.

Throughout these pages, you'll discover a range of delectable dishes that are simple to create, using healthful ingredients that are widely available at your local grocery shop. From vivid salads and hearty main courses to satisfying snacks and relaxing teas, each recipe is thoughtfully developed to help reduce inflammation and promote overall wellness. But this book is about more than simply recipes—it's about enabling you to take control of your health and create a deeper connection with the food you eat. You'll get practical suggestions, nutritional insights, and direction on how to navigate the grocery aisles with confidence, making it easier than ever to implement anti-inflammatory principles into your daily life.

Whether you're seeking relief from pain and discomfort, aiming to raise your energy levels, or simply wanting to feel your best from the inside out, the Anti-Inflammatory Diet Cookbook for Beginners is here to guide you every step of the way. So let's begin on this delectable trip together and explore the transformational power of food as medicine. Here's to healthy health and vitality!

Introduction to the Anti-Inflammatory Diet

The anti-inflammatory diet has attracted substantial interest in recent years for its possible health advantages in lowering inflammation throughout the body. Chronic inflammation is increasingly recognized as a contributing cause of several health conditions, including heart disease, diabetes, arthritis, and even certain malignancies. The concepts of the anti-inflammatory diet concentrate around ingesting foods that help decrease inflammation while avoiding those that may increase it.

Diet Principles:

1. **Emphasis on Whole Foods**: The core of the anti-inflammatory diet is whole, unprocessed foods. This includes fruits, legumes, nuts, vegetables, seeds, and whole grains. These foods are rich in vitamins, minerals, antioxidants, and phytonutrients, all of which have anti-inflammatory qualities.

2. **Omega-3 Fatty Acids**: Omega-3 fatty acids, found in fatty fish like salmon, mackerel, and sardines, as well as in walnuts, flaxseeds, and chia seeds, are known for their anti-inflammatory benefits. Incorporating these foods into the diet will help balance the body's omega-3 to omega-6 fatty acid ratio, which is vital for lowering inflammation.

3. **Healthy Fats**: In addition to omega-3 fatty acids, healthy fats such as those found in olive oil, avocados, and almonds are advised in the anti-inflammatory diet. These fats help reduce inflammation and supply critical nutrients for overall wellness.

4. **Limiting Inflammatory Meals**: Processed meals, refined carbs, sugary snacks and beverages, trans fats, and excessive consumption of red meat are all known to induce inflammation in the body. These foods should be reduced or avoided in an anti-inflammatory diet.

5. **Anti-Inflammatory Herbs and Spices**: Herbs and spices, including turmeric, ginger, garlic, and cinnamon, have significant anti-inflammatory

qualities. Incorporating these into cooking can boost the anti-inflammatory effects of meals.

Benefits of the Anti-Inflammatory Diet

1. **Reduced Inflammation**: By focusing on foods that assist in reducing inflammation and avoiding those that cause it, the anti-inflammatory diet can help reduce chronic inflammation in the body. This may lead to a decreased risk of inflammatory-related disorders.

2. **Improved Heart Health**: Many of the items emphasized in the anti-inflammatory diet, such as fruits, vegetables, and healthy fats, are also beneficial for heart health. By lowering inflammation and improving cardiovascular function, this diet can help minimize the risk of heart disease and enhance overall heart health.

3. **Weight Management:** The emphasis on complete, nutrient-dense foods in the anti-inflammatory diet can benefit weight management goals. These foods tend to be fewer in calories and higher in fiber, which can help induce satiety and minimize overeating.

4. **Enhanced Immune Function:** Chronic inflammation can weaken the immune system and make patients more susceptible to infections and illnesses. By lowering inflammation, the anti-inflammatory diet may help maintain immune function and enhance overall wellness.

5. **Improved Joint Health:** For those with inflammatory disorders such as arthritis, following an anti-inflammatory diet may help alleviate symptoms and improve joint health. Certain foods and nutrients present in this diet can help reduce inflammation and support joint function.

Overall, the anti-inflammatory diet offers a comprehensive approach to supporting health and well-being by focusing on nourishing, whole foods that support the body's natural anti-inflammatory processes. By embracing these dietary rules, individuals may experience a wide range of benefits that contribute to long-term health and vitality.

Tips for Beginners Getting Started With The Anti-Inflammatory Diet

Educate yourself: Take the time to study the concepts of the anti-inflammatory diet, including which foods to emphasize and which ones to minimize. Understanding why certain meals are helpful might help drive you to make healthier choices.

Start Gradually: Instead of trying to alter your entire diet overnight, start by making modest, doable modifications. For example, you may begin by integrating one new anti-inflammatory ingredient into your meals each day or week.

Focus on entire foods: base your meals around entire, unprocessed foods such as fruits, vegetables, whole grains, nuts, seeds, and legumes. These meals are rich in minerals and antioxidants that help reduce inflammation.

Experiment with Recipes: Explore new recipes that incorporate anti-inflammatory components. There are many cookbooks, websites, and apps dedicated to healthy eating that can provide inspiration and assistance.

Include Omega-3 Fatty Acids: Incorporate sources of omega-3 fatty acids into your diet, such as fatty fish (salmon, mackerel, and sardines), walnuts, flaxseeds, and chia seeds. These lipids have potent anti-inflammatory properties.

Use Healthy Fats: Replace unhealthy fats like trans fats and saturated fats with healthier ones such as olive oil, avocado oil, almonds, and seeds. These fats can help reduce inflammation and enhance general wellness.

Add Anti-Inflammatory Herbs and Spices: Experiment with herbs and spices like turmeric, ginger, garlic, and cinnamon, which have significant anti-inflammatory qualities. Incorporating these into your cooking can increase the flavor of your dishes while improving their health benefits.

Read Labels: Pay attention to food labels and ingredient lists when shopping at supermarkets. Avoid goods that have added sugars, processed grains, trans fats, and artificial additives, as these can increase inflammation.

Stay Hydrated: Drink a lot of water throughout the day to stay hydrated. Limit consumption of sugary beverages and choose water, herbal teas, or infused water with slices of fruits or herbs for flavor.

Be Mindful of Portions: While focusing on nutrient-dense foods is vital, it's equally essential to be mindful of portion sizes to maintain a healthy balance. Pay attention to hunger and fullness signs to prevent overeating.

Plan Ahead: Take time to plan your meals and snacks for the week ahead. This can help you make healthier choices and avoid grabbing for handy but less nutritious options when you're hungry.

Listen to your body: Pay attention to how different foods make you feel. Notice any changes in energy levels, digestion, or overall well-being when you start introducing more anti-inflammatory foods into your diet.

Don't compare your body with others because you are different, so stay positive. It may take some time to find the appropriate balance of foods that work best for you and your specific needs. Be gentle with yourself, and reward your progress along the way.

How To Use This Book

Using a book on the anti-inflammatory diet may be an overwhelming resource for learning more about the concepts of the diet, discovering new recipes, and receiving practical suggestions for incorporating anti-inflammatory foods into your lifestyle. Here's some advice on how to efficiently use a book on the anti-inflammatory diet:

1. **Read the Introduction and Overview:** Start by reading the introduction and overview sections of the book. This will offer you an overview of the ideas underlying the anti-inflammatory diet, including why particular foods are healthy and how they can help reduce inflammation in the body.

2. **Explore the Food Lists:** Many anti-inflammatory diet publications contain lists of foods to promote and foods to limit or avoid. Take the time to familiarize yourself with these lists, as they will act as a reference for choosing meal selections when following the plan.

3. **Browse the Recipes:** One of the highlights of many anti-inflammatory diet books is the array of recipes included. Take some time to look through the recipes and bookmark ones that appeal to you. Look for recipes that showcase full,

unprocessed meals and use anti-inflammatory components like fruits, vegetables, herbs, spices, nuts, seeds, and healthy fats.

4. **Build a Meal Plan:** Use the recipes in the book to build a meal plan for the week ahead. Consider aspects such as your schedule, food habits, and any specific health goals you have. Planning your meals in advance will help you stay organized and ensure that you have the appropriate items on hand. There is a simple meal plan that has been created for you in this book.

5. **Try New Ingredients and Techniques:** As you explore the recipes in the book, don't be hesitant to try new ingredients and cooking techniques. Experimenting with different flavors and cooking methods can help keep your meals interesting and enjoyable.

6. **Modify Recipes to Suit Your Preferences:** Feel free to modify the recipes in the book to suit your taste preferences and nutritional demands. You can alter ingredients, portion quantities, and cooking methods as needed to make the recipes work for you.

7. **Keep Track of Your Success:** Use the book as a tool for documenting your success on the anti-inflammatory diet. Keep a journal of the meals you eat, how you feel after eating them, and any changes you see in your overall health and well-being.

8. **Refer Back for Inspiration:** Keep the book nearby for continuing inspiration and encouragement. Refer back to it whenever you need ideas for meals or recommendations for staying on track with the anti-inflammatory diet.

9. **Share with Others:** If you find the book helpful, consider sharing it with friends or family members who may also benefit from learning about the anti-inflammatory diet. Sharing resources and support might help you stay motivated and accountable on your road towards better health.

By following these steps, you may effectively use a book on the anti-inflammatory diet as a helpful resource for enhancing your health and well-being through nourishing, anti-inflammatory foods and dishes.

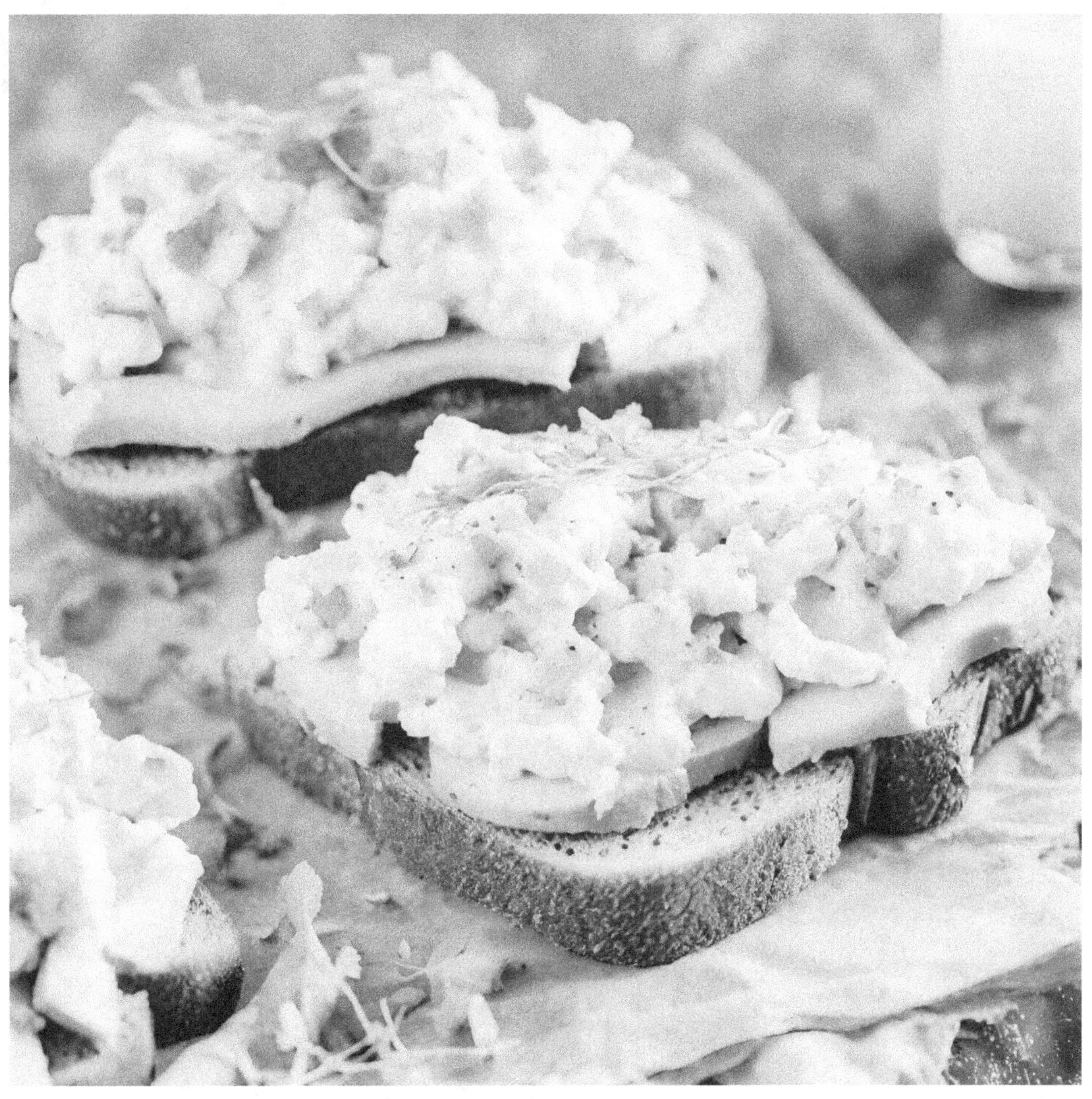

BREAKFAST RECIPES

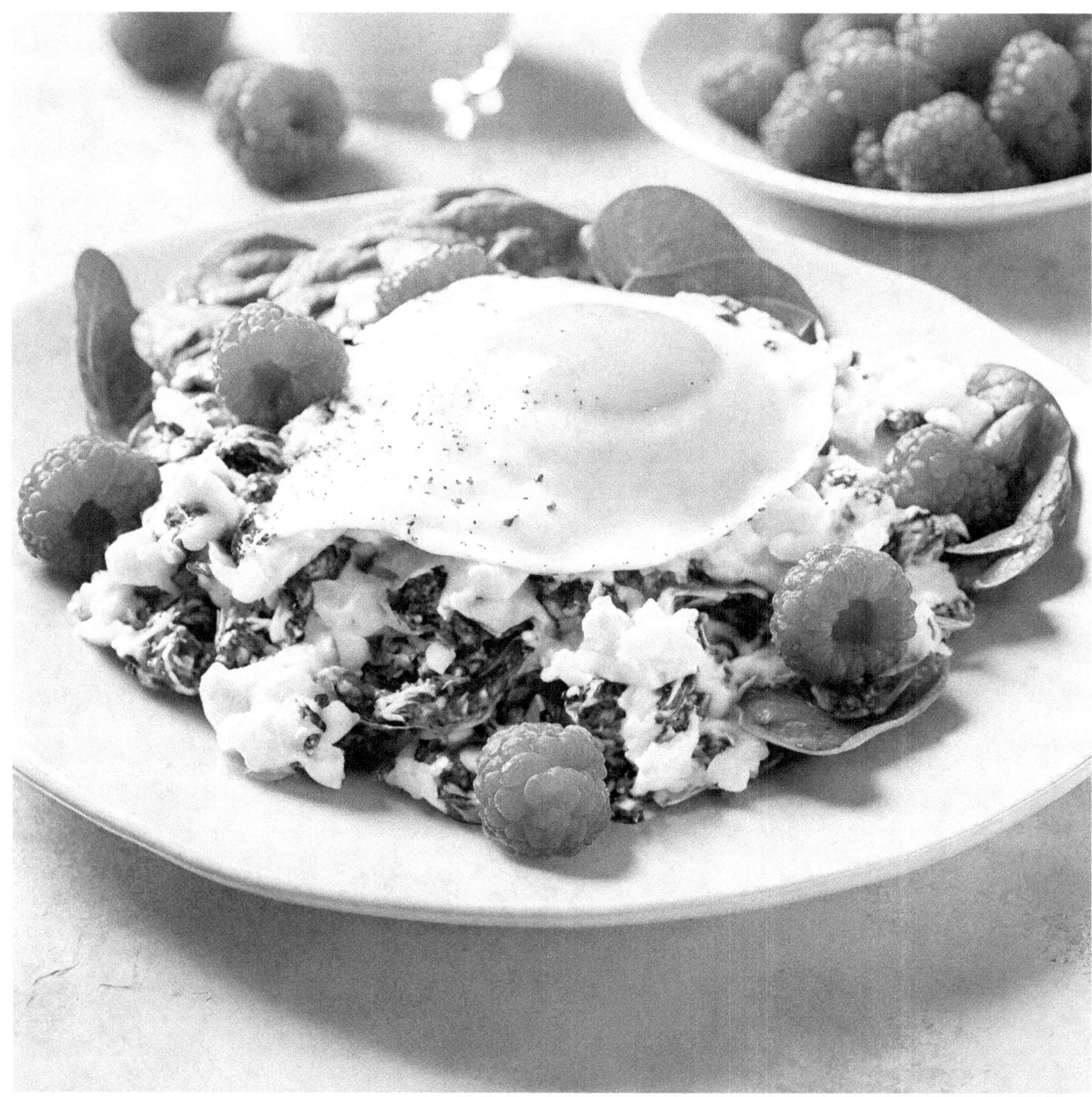

Spinach and Egg Scramble with Raspberries

Nutritional Facts: 296 Calories, 16g fat, 21g carbs, 18g Protein

Prep Time: 10 minutes, Total Time: 10 minutes, Servings: 1

Ingredient

1 teaspoon canola oil
1 ½ cups of baby spinach (1 1/2 ounces)
2 big eggs, lightly beaten
Pinch of kosher salt
Pinch of ground pepper
1 slice whole-grain bread, toasted

½ cup fresh raspberries

Directions

Heat oil over medium-high heat in a nonstick skillet. Add spinach and heat until wilted, stirring constantly for 1 to 2 minutes. Transfer the spinach to a dish. Wipe the pan clean, set it over medium heat, and add the eggs. Cook, tossing once or twice to ensure consistent cooking, until just set, 1 to 2 minutes. Stir in the spinach, salt, and pepper. Serve the scramble with toast and strawberries

Egg Salad Avocado Toast

Nutrition Facts: 230 Calories, 14g fat, 17g carbs,11g Protein

Prep Time: 5 minutes, Total Time: 5 minutes, Servings: 1

Ingredients:

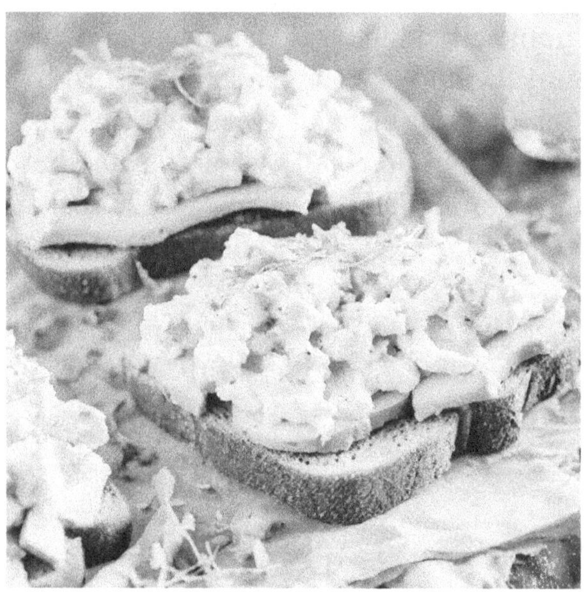

¼ avocado
1 tablespoon celery
½ teaspoon lemon juice
½ teaspoon spicy sauce

Pinch of salt
1 sliced hard-boiled egg
1 piece of whole-wheat bread

Directions

Mash avocado with celery, lemon juice, spicy sauce, and salt in a small bowl. Mix in a hard-boiled egg. Spread it on toast.

Smoked Salmon and Cream Cheese Omelet

Nutrition Facts: 254 Calories, 19g fat, 3g carbs, 17g Protein

Cook Time: 15 minutes, Total Time: 15 minutes, Servings: 1

Ingredients

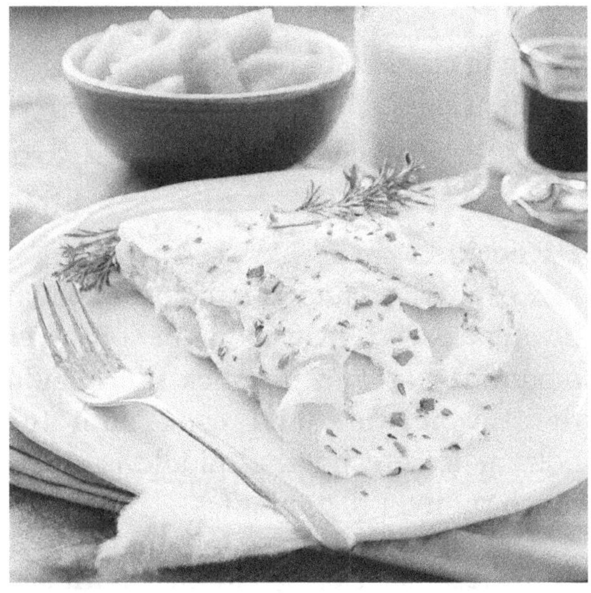

2 big eggs
1 teaspoon reduced-fat milk or water
⅛ teaspoon of ground pepper
Pinch of salt
1 teaspoon butter
2 teaspoons chopped smoked salmon
1 tablespoon cream cheese, softened, or crumbled feta
1 tablespoon coarsely chopped red onion
1 ½ tablespoons of chopped fresh dill

Directions

Whisk eggs, milk (or water), pepper, and salt in a small bowl. Melt butter in a small nonstick skillet over medium-low heat, turning the pan to make sure the entire bottom is coated. Add the egg mixture and simmer for 1 minute without stirring.

Sprinkle salmon, cheese, onion, and dill over one half of the eggs. Cook for 1 minute. Using a flexible spatula, elevate the naked side to let raw eggs from the middle flow underneath; you may need to tilt the pan slightly.

Continue lifting in different locations until there's hardly any raw egg on top. Cook for 2 minutes more. Using the spatula, flip the bare side over the filling, fold the omelet in half, and cook for 1 minute. (If the eggs are starting to brown, decrease the heat.) Carefully flip the omelet over and cook for 1 minute more.

Serve immediately, topped with additional dill and pepper, if desired.

Avocado and Kale Omelet

Nutrition Facts: 339 Calories, 28g fat, 9g carbs, 15g Protein

Prep Time: 10 minutes, Total Time: 10 minutes, Servings: 1

Ingredients

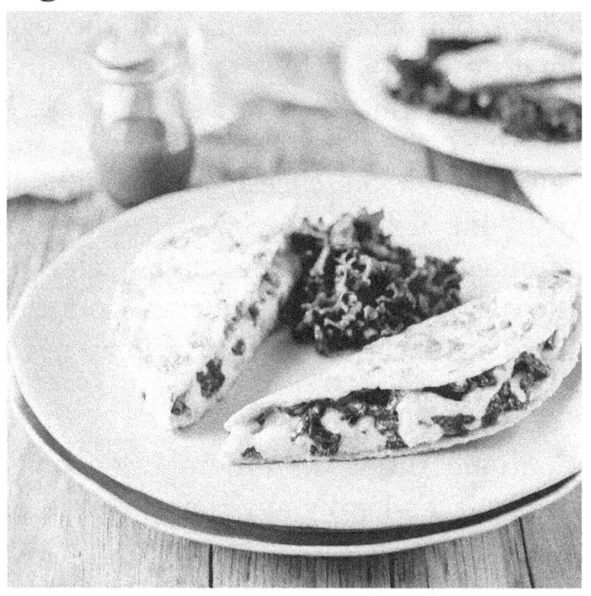

2 big eggs
1 teaspoon low-fat milk
Pinch of salt

2 tablespoons extra-virgin olive oil
1 cup chopped kale
1 tablespoon of lime juice
1 tablespoon chopped fresh cilantro
1 teaspoon of unsalted sunflower seeds

Pinch of crushed red pepper
Pinch of salt

¼ avocado, sliced

Directions
Mix eggs with salt and milk in a medium bowl. Heat 1 teaspoon of oil over medium heat in a nonstick skillet. Add the egg mixture and cook until the bottom is set and the middle is still a touch runny, 1 to 2 minutes.

Flip the omelet over and heat until set, about 30 seconds more. Transfer to a plate.

Toss kale with the remaining 1 teaspoon oil, lime juice, cilantro, sunflower seeds, smashed red pepper, and a sprinkle of salt. Top the omelet with the kale salad and avocado.

Spinach & Feta Scrambled Egg Pitas

Nutrition Facts: 303 Calories, 16g fat, 21g carbs, 20g Protein

Prep Time: 15 minutes, Total Time: 15 minutes, Servings: 4

Ingredients

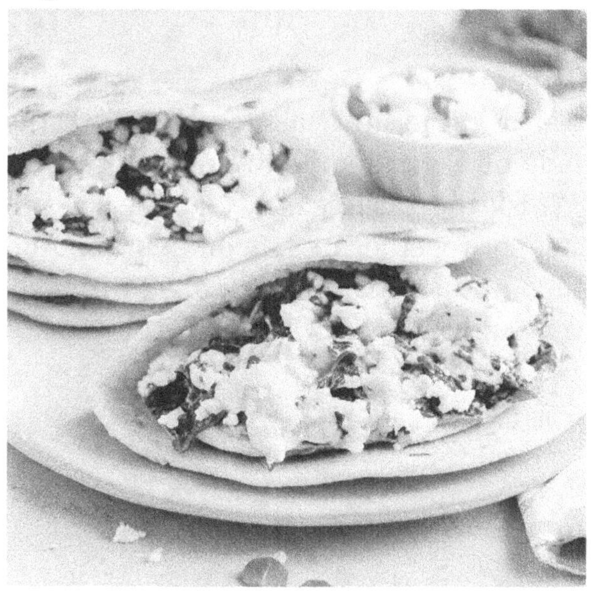

1 tablespoon extra-virgin olive oil

1 (10-ounce) block of frozen chopped spinach, thawed, drained, and squeezed dry

Pinch salt
8 big eggs, beaten

¼ cup finely shredded feta cheese
Freshly ground pepper, to taste

8 teaspoons of sun-dried tomato tapenade or sun-dried tomato pesto

4 whole-wheat pitas (5-inch), split in half, warmed if desired

Directions
In a large nonstick skillet, heat the oil over medium heat. Add spinach and salt and boil until steaming hot, stirring periodically.

Add eggs and cook, turning the eggs as they set, until they form soft curds and are just wet, 4 to 5 minutes.

Add feta and pepper and simmer until set. Put two tablespoons of tapenade (or pesto) inside each pita pocket. Distribute the mixture of eggs among the pitas.

Baby Kale Breakfast Salad with Smoked Trout and Avocado

Nutrition Facts: 275 Calories, 23g fat, 9g carbs, 10g Protein

Cook Time: 15 minutes, Total Time: 15 minutes, Servings: 1

Ingredients
1 teaspoon minced garlic
Pinch of salt
1 tablespoon extra-virgin olive oil
2 teaspoons red-wine vinegar
Pinch of pepper
3 cups of lightly packed baby kale
¼ cup flaky smoked trout

¼ firm ripe avocado, cut or diced
1 tablespoon coarsely chopped red onion

Directions
Mash garlic and salt together with the side of a chef's knife to produce a paste. Whisk the garlic paste, oil, vinegar, and pepper together in a medium basin. Add kale; toss to coat. Serve topped with fish, avocado, and red onion.

Avocado and Arugula Omelet

Nutrition Facts: 344 Calories, 28g fat, 7g carbs, 17g protein

Prep Time: 10 minutes, Total Time: 10 minutes, Servings: 1

Ingredients
2 big eggs
1 teaspoon low-fat milk
⅛ teaspoon salt, divided
2 teaspoons extra-virgin olive oil, divided

½ cup arugula
1 teaspoon of lemon juice
¼ avocado, diced
2 tablespoons plain whole-milk Greek yogurt

Directions

Beat eggs with milk and a touch of salt in a small bowl. In a small nonstick skillet, heat up 1 teaspoon of oil over medium heat. Add the egg mixture and cook until the bottom is set and the middle is still a touch runny, 1 to 2 minutes.

Flip the omelet over and heat until set, about 30 seconds more. Transfer to a plate.

Toss arugula with the remaining 1 teaspoon oil and lemon juice in a small bowl. Top the omelet with avocado, yogurt, the arugula, and the remaining pinch of salt.

Smoked Trout and Spinach Scrambled Eggs

Nutrition Facts: 243 Calories, 17g fat, 4g carbs, 19g Protein

Prep Time: 15 minutes, Total Time: 15 minutes, Servings: 2

Ingredients

4 big eggs
2 tablespoons of reduced-fat milk
¼ teaspoon powdered pepper

Pinch of salt
2 teaspoons of grapeseed oil or avocado oil
2 teaspoons of finely chopped shallot
½ cup boned and flakes smoked trout (1 1/2 ounces)
1 cup chopped spinach

Directions

Whisk eggs, milk, pepper, and salt in a medium bowl until pale yellow throughout.

In a medium nonstick skillet, heat the oil over medium heat. Add shallot and cook, stirring, for 1 to 2 minutes, or until beginning to brown.

Add the egg mixture and lower the heat to medium-low. Cook, undisturbed, until the edges start to harden, about 30 seconds. Sprinkle trout over the eggs.

Using a rubber spatula, gently push and fold the eggs until frothy and just set, 2 to 4 minutes. Stir in spinach. Remove from heat, cover, and let stand until the spinach is just wilted, 1 to 2 minutes.

Breakfast Beans with Microwave-Poached Egg

Nutrition Facts: 364 Calories, 20g fat, 32g carbs, 16g Protein

Prep Time: 15 minutes, Total Time: 15 minutes, Servings: 2

Ingredients
2 tablespoons canola oil

¼ cup sliced red bell pepper
2 chopped onions, whites, and greens separated
½ teaspoon ground cumin
¾ cup rinsed canned low-sodium black beans
½ cup boiled barley
½ cup low-sodium chicken broth or vegetarian broth
⅛ teaspoon salt
⅛ teaspoon spicy sauce
1 cup of water, divided
1 teaspoon distilled white vinegar, split 2 big eggs, and divide
2 tablespoons of shredded pepper Jack cheese

½ avocado, sliced
2 teaspoons roughly chopped fresh cilantro

Directions
In a medium skillet, heat the oil over medium heat. Add bell pepper, scallion whites, and cumin; simmer, turning regularly, until softened, 1 to 2 minutes.

Add beans, boiled barley, broth, and salt. It takes three to five minutes of cooking to absorb most of the liquid. Stir in the scallion greens and spicy sauce. Divide between two bowls.

Place 1/2 cup water and 1/2 teaspoon . vinegar in a microwave-safe small bowl. Carefully crack one egg into the water so it is completely submerged.

Cover with a microwave-safe plate and microwave on high until the egg white is firm and the yolk is still somewhat runny, about 1 minute. (If required, continue to microwave, checking every 10 seconds.)

Remove the egg with a slotted spoon, pat it dry, and place it on top of the bean mixture in a bowl.

Continue using the remaining 1/2 cup and 1/2 tsp of water, vinegar, and egg.Top each bowl with 1 Tbsp. cheese and 1/4 avocado. Sprinkle with cilantro, if desired.

Avocado and Smoked Salmon Omelet

Nutrition Facts: 323 Calories, 25g fat, 5g carbs, 19g Protein

Prep Time: 10 minutes, Total Time: 10 minutes, Servings: 1

Ingredient

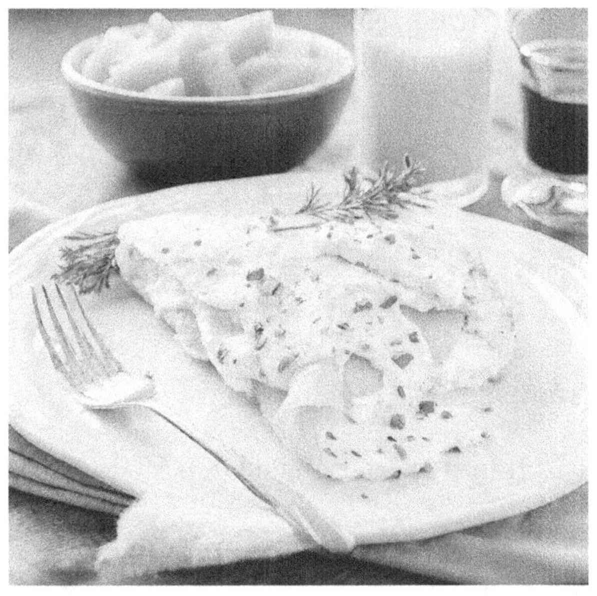

2 big eggs
1 teaspoon low-fat milk
Pinch of salt
1 teaspoon extra-virgin olive oil

¼ avocado, sliced
1 ounce of smoked salmon
1 tablespoon chopped fresh basil

Directions

In a small bowl, beat eggs with milk and salt. In a small nonstick skillet, heat up one teaspoon of oil over medium heat.

Add the egg mixture and cook until the bottom is set and the middle is still a touch runny, 1 to 2 minutes. Flip the omelet over and heat until set, about 30 seconds more.

Transfer to a plate. Top with avocado, salmon, and basil. Drizzle with the remaining 1/2 teaspoon of oil.

Avocado-Egg Toast

Nutrition Facts: 271 Calories., 18g of fat, 18g of carbs, and 12g of protein.

Cook Time: 5 minutes, Total time: 5 minutes., Servings: One.

Ingredients:

¼ avocado.
1/4 teaspoon of ground pepper
⅛ teaspoon garlic powder.
1 slice of toasted whole wheat bread.
1 large, fried egg
1 teaspoon of Sriracha (optional)
1 tablespoon sliced scallions (optional)

Directions

In a small bowl, combine the avocado, pepper, and garlic powder and gently mash.

Top the toast with the avocado mixture and a fried egg. Garnish with Sriracha and scallions, if desired.

Smoked Salmon Scrambled Eggs

Nutrition Facts: 205 Calories., 13g fat, 2g carbs., 19g protein.

Prep Time: 10 minutes., Total time: 10 minutes., Servings: One.

Ingredients

Two huge eggs.
1 ounce smoked salmon, diced.
2 teaspoons of reduced-fat cream cheese.
One scallion, sliced
1 teaspoon capers, washed

Directions

In a small bowl, lightly beat the eggs until well blended. Stir in the smoked salmon, cream cheese, scallions, and capers.

Coat a small nonstick skillet with cooking spray and set it over medium heat. Add the egg mixture and heat, stirring frequently, until scrambled, about 3 minutes.

Beans on Toast

Nutrition Facts: 183 Calories, 4g fat, 28g carbs., 5g protein.

Cook Time: 20 minutes., Total time: 20 minutes., Servings: four

Ingredients:
1 tablespoon of unsalted butter.
3 cups of thinly cut cremini mushrooms.
1 ½ tablespoons low-sodium Worcestershire sauce
2 tsp. tomato paste
¾ teaspoon chili powder.
¼ teaspoon salt
1 (13.7-ounce) can of baked beans in tomato sauce (such as Heinz).
Four slices of multigrain bread, toasted
1 tablespoon chopped fresh flat-leaved parsley.

Directions
Over medium-high heat, melt the butter in a large saucepan. Add the mushrooms and simmer, stirring periodically, for about 5 minutes, or until tender.

Reduce the heat to medium; mix in Worcestershire sauce, tomato paste, chili powder, and salt until thoroughly combined.

Cook, stirring periodically, until the liquid has evaporated and the mushrooms have turned golden brown, about 5 minutes.

Reduce the heat to low and cook, stirring periodically, until the beans are well heated, about 3 to 5 minutes.

Spread 1/2 cup of the bean mixture over each slice of toast, and garnish with parsley.

Feta, Egg, and Olive Pita.

Nutrition Facts: 287 Calories., 13g fat, 27g carbohydrates, 16g protein.

Cook Time: 10 minutes., Total time: 10 minutes., Servings: One.

Ingredients
2 tablespoons whole-milk plain Greek yogurt
½ whole wheat pita and ¼ cup baby arugula.
2 tablespoons of halved cherry tomatoes.
1 big, poached egg
Three pitted Kalamata olives, diced
1 tablespoon of crumbled feta cheese.
¼ teaspoon Za'atar

Directions
Spread yogurt inside the pita. Fill each pita with arugula, tomatoes, a poached egg, olives, and feta. Sprinkle with Za'atar.

Chickpea and Kale Toast.

Nutrition Facts: 397 Calories., 18g fat, 40g carbs., 19g protein.

Cook Time: 10 minutes., Total time: 10 minutes., Servings: Two.

Ingredients
1 tablespoon of extra virgin olive oil.
8 cups chopped kale.
2 garlic cloves, minced
1 cup of washed, salt-free canned chickpeas
A pinch of ground pepper.
2 slices of whole-grain bread, toasted
1/2 cup crumbled feta cheese.

Directions
Over medium-high heat, heat the oil in a large skillet. Cook the greens and garlic, stirring regularly, until tender, about 4 minutes.

Stir in the chickpeas, salt, and pepper. Evenly divide the mixture between the toast slices. Sprinkle with feta.

Berry-Orange Chia Pudding

Nutrition Facts: 188 Calories., 9g fat, 26g carbs., 4g protein.

Cook Time: 10 minutes, Total time: 20 minutes, Servings: 4

Ingredients
1 (14-ounce) can of coconut milk
1 cup mixed berries.
1/2 cup orange juice.
1/2 cup chia seeds.
2 teaspoons of pure maple syrup.

Directions
Blend the coconut milk, berries, and orange juice in a blender until smooth. Transfer it to a container.

Combine the chia seeds with maple syrup. Cover and refrigerate overnight.

Rosemary, Tomato, and Feta Egg Sandwiches.

Nutrition Facts: 242 Calories., 12g fat, 25g carbs., 13g protein.

Prep Time: 5 minutes., Cook time: 15 minutes., Total time: 20 minutes., Servings: 4

Ingredients
4 Multigrain Sandwich Thins
4 tsp. olive oil
1 tablespoon clipped fresh rosemary or 1/2 teaspoon dried rosemary, crushed
4 eggs
2 cups of fresh baby spinach leaves.
1 medium tomato, sliced into eight thin slices.
4 tablespoons of reduced-fat feta cheese.
⅛ teaspoon kosher salt.
Freshly ground black pepper.

Directions
Preheat the oven to 375°F. Split the sandwich thin and brush the sliced sides with 2 tablespoons of olive oil.

Place on a rimmed baking sheet and bake for approximately 5 minutes, or until the edges are light golden and crispy.

Meanwhile, in a large pan, heat the remaining 2 tablespoons of olive oil and rosemary over medium-high heat. Break one egg at a time into the skillet.

Cook for approximately a minute, or until the whites are set but the yolks remain liquid. Break the yolks with a spatula. Flip the eggs and cook on the other side until done. Remove from heat.

Place the bottom half of the toasted sandwich thin on four serving plates. Divide the spinach between the sandwiches thin on the plates.

Top each with two tomato slices, an egg, and one tablespoon of feta cheese. Sprinkle it with salt and pepper. Top with the remaining thin sandwich halves.

Skillet Eggs with Tomatillos and Spinach.

Nutrition Facts: 210 Calories., 15g fat, 10g carbs., 11g protein.

Prep Time: 30 minutes., Total time: 30 minutes., Servings: 4

Ingredients
2 tablespoons extra virgin olive oil
1 cup cut spring onions or scallions.
2 cloves of garlic, coarsely chopped
1 finely chopped jalapeño or serrano pepper.
1 teaspoon ground cumin.
8 ounces of diced tomatillos or green tomatoes.
8 cups of chopped mature spinach.
¼ cup water
1/2 cup chopped flat-leaf parsley.
1/4 cup chopped fresh cilantro.
¼ cup chopped fresh mint.
¼ teaspoon salt
Four big eggs.
1/4 cup crumbled feta cheese.
Garnish with cracked pepper and harissa.

Directions
Over medium heat, heat the oil in a medium skillet. Cook, turning occasionally, until spring onions (or scallions) are soft but not browned, about 1 to 2 minutes.

Cook garlic, jalapeño (or serrano), and cumin until aromatic (approximately 30 seconds).

Stir in the tomatillos (or green tomatoes) and simmer for approximately 5 minutes, stirring periodically, until they begin to break down.

Stir in the spinach and water; simmer for approximately 1 minute, or until wilted. Stir in the parsley, cilantro, mint, and salt.

Crack eggs over the veggies. Cook for 3 to 5 minutes, covered, over medium-low heat, until the whites set.

Remove from the fire and sprinkle with feta; cover and set aside for 2 minutes. Garnish with cracked pepper and harissa, if preferred.

Spinach and Egg Sweet Potato Toast

Nutrition Facts: 124 Calories., 5g fat, 12g carbs., 9g protein.

Preparation Time: 10 minutes, Total time: 20 minutes., Servings: One.

Ingredients

1 big slice of sweet potato (1/4 inch thick).
⅓ cup cooked spinach.
One big egg, fried or poached
1/2 teaspoon sliced fresh chives.
½ teaspoon of spicy sauce.

Directions

Toast sweet potatoes in a toaster or toaster oven for 12 to 15 minutes, or until they are just cooked through and beginning to color. Garnish with spinach, eggs, chives, and spicy sauce.

Two-Ingredient Banana Pancakes

Nutrition Facts:124 Calories., 5g fat, 14g carbs., 7g protein.

Cook Time: 15 minutes., Total time: 15 minutes., Servings: 2

Ingredients
Two huge eggs.
1 medium banana.

Directions
Blend the eggs and banana until smooth. Lightly oil a big nonstick pan and place it over medium heat.

Drop 4 mounds of batter onto the pan, using 2 teaspoons for each pancake.

Cook until bubbles develop on the surface and the edges seem dry, about 2 to 4 minutes.

Flip the pancakes carefully with a thin spatula and cook for another 1 to 2 minutes, or until the bottom is golden.

Move the pancakes to a platter. Lightly oil the pan again, then repeat with the remaining batter.

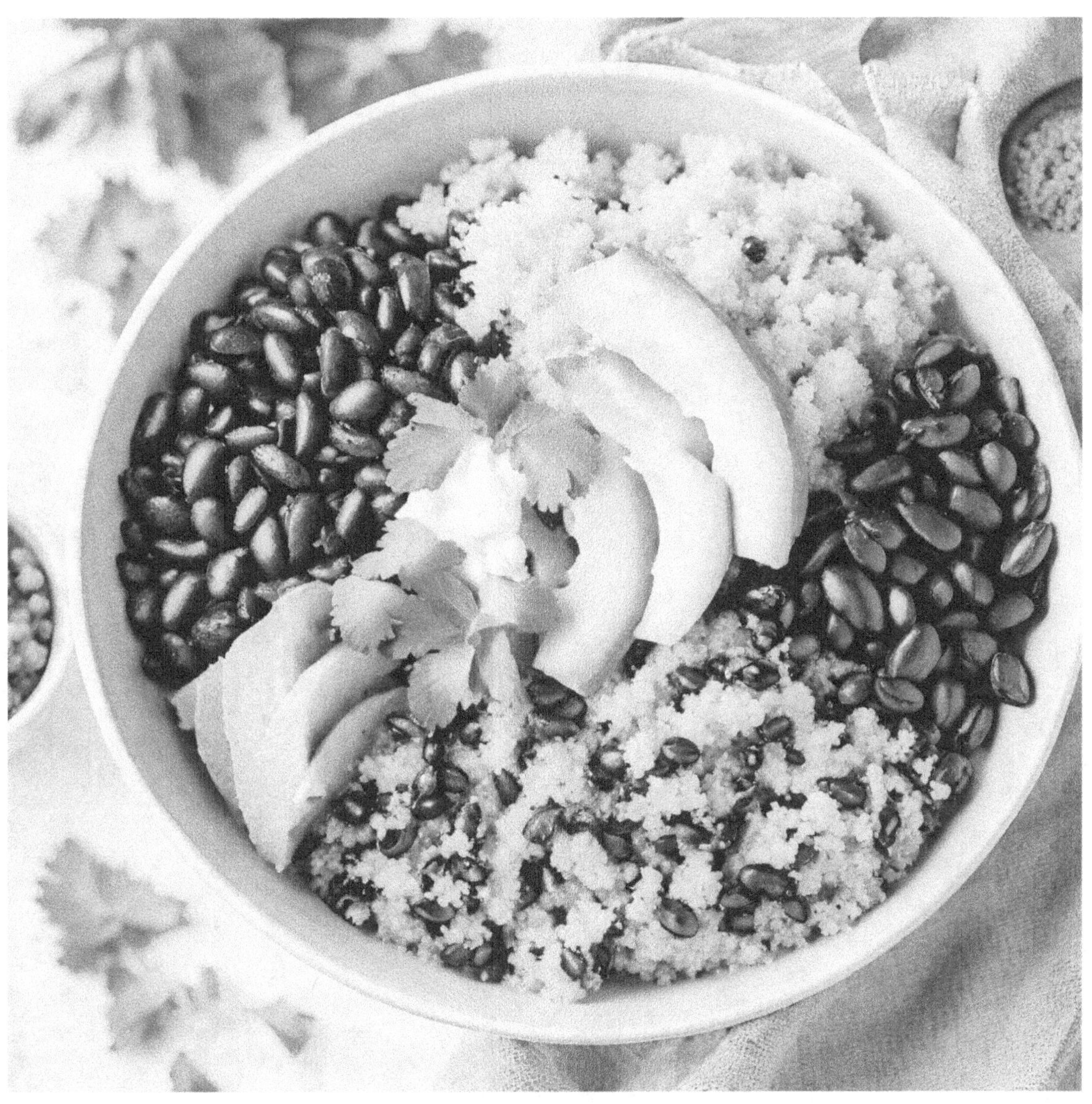

LUNCH RECIPES

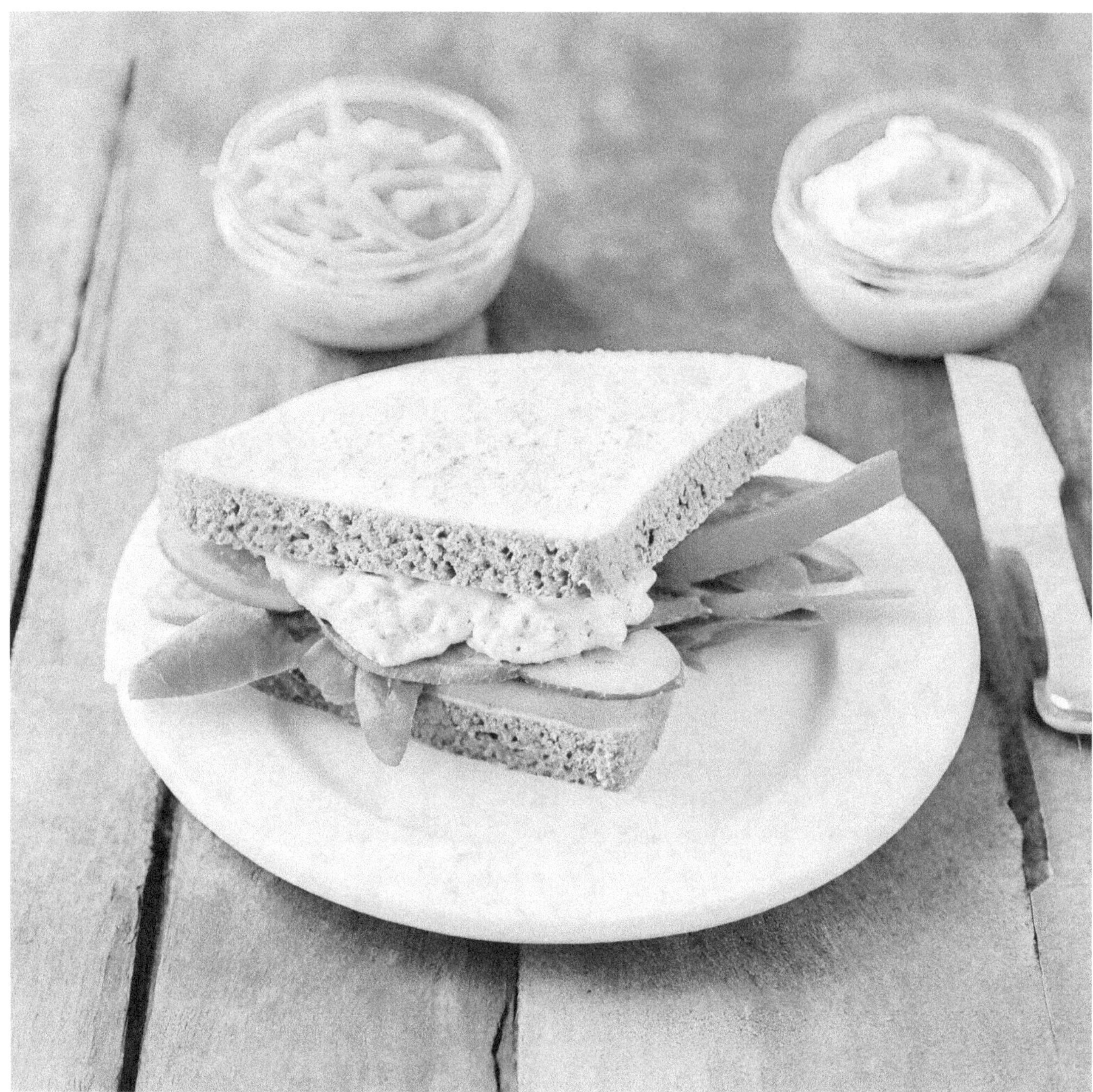

Veggie and Hummus Sandwich.

Nutrition Facts: 325 Calories, 14g fat, 40g carbs., 13g protein.

Cook Time: 10 minutes., Total time: 10 minutes., Servings: One.

Ingredients

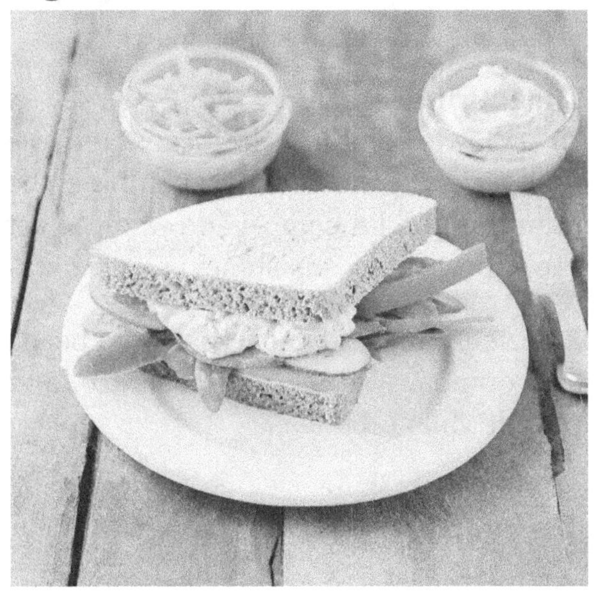

2 pieces of whole-grain bread.
3 tablespoons hummus,

¼ avocado (mashed).
1/2 cup mixed salad greens.
¼ medium red bell pepper

¼ cup sliced cucumber.
¼ cup grated carrot

Directions

Spread avocado on one slice of bread and hummus on the other. Fill the sandwich with greens, bell peppers, cucumbers, and carrots. Slice in half and serve.

Black Bean-Quinoa Bowl

Nutrition Facts: 500 Calories, 16g fat, 74g carbs., 20g protein.

Preparation Time: 10 minutes, Total time: 10 minutes., Servings: One.

Ingredients:

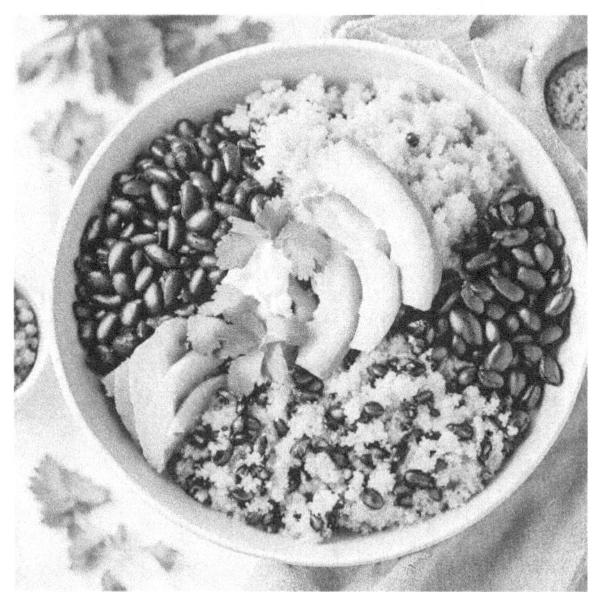

¾ cup canned, rinsed black beans.
⅔ cup cooked quinoa

¼ cup hummus.
1 tablespoon of lime juice.
¼ medium avocado, diced
Three tablespoons. Pico de Gallo

2 tablespoons of chopped fresh cilantro.

Directions

In a bowl, combine the beans and the quinoa. In a small bowl, combine the hummus and lime juice; add water to get the appropriate consistency.

Drizzle hummus dressing over the beans and quinoa. Add avocado, cilantro, and pico de gallo on top.

Chickpea Tuna Salad.

Nutrition Facts: 357 Calories, 19g fat, 23g carbohydrates.,21g protein.

Cook Time: 20 minutes., Total time: 20 minutes., Servings: 4

Ingredients

2 teaspoons of lemon juice.
1 tablespoon of nonpareil capers, washed and diced
1 tablespoon finely chopped shallot

¼ teaspoon salt

¼ teaspoon ground pepper.
One (15-ounce) can of no-salted chickpeas, washed
1 (6.7 ounce) jar of oil-packed tuna (drained)
1 cup halved cherry tomatoes.
1 cup of finely sliced English cucumber.
1/2 cup crumbled feta cheese.
2 tablespoons of chopped fresh dill.
Three tablespoons of extra-virgin olive oil
3 cups baby spinach.

Directions

Combine lemon juice, capers, shallots, salt, and pepper in a large bowl. Leave it for a duration of five minutes. Meanwhile, combine chickpeas, tuna, tomatoes, cucumber, feta, and dill in a large bowl.

Whisk the oil into the lemon juice mixture until thoroughly combined. To coat the chickpeas, add roughly 5 tablespoons of the dressing.

Toss the spinach with the remaining dressing in a large bowl until well coated. Divide the spinach evenly among four dishes and top each with 1 1/4 cups of chickpea mixture. Serve immediately.

Lemony Lentil Salad with Feta.

Nutrition Facts: 280 Calories., 16g fat, 24g carbs., 13g protein.

Cook time: 30 minutes., Total time: 30 minutes., Servings: 6.

Ingredients:

⅓ cup lemon juice.
⅓ cup chopped fresh dill

2 teaspoons Dijon mustard

¼ teaspoon salt (or to taste).
⅓ cup extra virgin olive oil.
Freshly ground pepper to taste.
Two washed 15-ounce cans of lentils or three cups of cooked brown or green lentils

One cup (about four ounces) of crumbled feta cheese

1 medium red bell pepper, seeded and chopped (about 1 cup).
1 cup chopped, seedless cucumber
1/2 cup finely chopped red onion.

Directions

Combine lemon juice, dill, mustard, salt, and pepper in a large mixing basin. Gradually whisk in the oil. Toss in the lentils, feta, bell pepper, cucumber, and onion until coated.

Loaded Cucumber and Avocado Sandwich.

Nutrition Facts: 403 Calories, 23g fat, 35g carbs., 17g protein.

Cook Time: 10 minutes., Total time: 10 minutes., Servings: One.

Ingredients

3 tablespoons of shredded extra-sharp cheddar cheese.
2 tablespoons ricotta cheese.
4 tablespoons of coarsely sliced chives
2 tablespoons of lemon juice.
Grind pepper to taste.

2 slices of whole wheat sandwich bread, gently toasted.
⅓ cup finely sliced cucumber.
1/4 cup finely sliced red bell pepper.
⅓ avocado, sliced

Directions

In a small bowl, combine cheddar, ricotta, chives, lemon juice, salt, and pepper. Spread half of the mixture on each slice of bread. Layer one piece with cucumber, pepper, and avocado, then top with the second slice, spread side down.

Avocado Tuna Spinach Salad

Nutrition Facts: 432 Calories, 32g fat, 17g carbs., 20g protein.

Cook Time: 10 minutes, Total time: 10 minutes.Servings: One.

Ingredients

½ (5-ounce) can of water-packed tuna
¼ cup diced avocado
1/4 cup halved cherry tomatoes.
1 ½ teaspoons poppy seed dressing.
1 tablespoon of chopped red onion.
1 tablespoon of extra virgin olive oil.
2 cups baby spinach.
1 tablespoon of sunflower seeds.

Directions

In a medium bowl, combine tuna, avocado, tomatoes, seasoning, onion, and oil. Serve over spinach, and garnish with sunflower seeds.

Vegan Burrito Bowls with Cauliflower Rice.

Nutrition Facts: 298 calories, 20g fat, 15g carbs., 15g protein.

Prep Time: 25 minutes., Total time: 25 minutes., Servings: 4

Ingredients

Tofu crumbles

1 (12-ounce) box of frozen riced cauliflower.
4 tsp. olive oil

1 teaspoon taco seasoning (no salt added)
1 cup finely sliced red cabbage.
1 cup chopped avocado.
1/2 cup pico de gallo o salsa.
1/4 cup chopped fresh cilantro.

Directions

Prepare the tofu crumbles as indicated. While the tofu crumbles cook, make the riced cauliflower according to the package directions. Toss in oil and taco seasoning.

Divide the cauliflower into four single-serving containers with lids.Add 1/4 cup of avocado and cabbage, 1/2 cup of beefless ground beef, 2 teaspoons of pico de gallo (or salsa), and 1 tablespoon of cilantro on top.

Seal the containers and chill until ready to consume.

Arugula and Cucumber Salad with Tuna

Nutrition Facts: 232 Calories., 13g fat, 2g carbs., 26g protein.

Cook Time: 15 minutes., Total time: 15 minutes., Servings: 4

Ingredients:

3 tablespoons chopped fresh basil.
1 tablespoon white wine vinegar.
1 ½ teaspoon lemon juice.
½ teaspoon salt.
Three tablespoons of extra-virgin olive oil
¾ cup thinly sliced celery

¾ cup sliced Persian or English cucumber.
1 (5 oz.) packet of baby arugula
8 pitted Castelvetrano olives, quartered

(approx. 1/3 cup)
Two (6.7-ounce) packets. Tuna filets in water with no salt added, drained

Directions

Combine the basil, vinegar, lemon juice, and salt in a large bowl. Add the oil and stir to mix. Toss in celery, cucumber, arugula, and olives.

Divide among four bowls, and top with flaked tuna.

Mediterranean Tuna and Spinach Salad.

Nutrition Facts: 376 Calories, 21g fat, 26g carbs, 26g protein.

Cook time: 10 minutes., Total time: 10 minutes., Servings: one

Ingredients:

1 ½ teaspoons tahini

1 ½ tablespoons lemon juice.
1 ½ teaspoons of water.
One 5-ounce can of chunk light tuna in water that has been drained
Four Kalamata olives, pitted and chopped
2 tablespoons of feta cheese.
2 tablespoons of parsley

2 cups baby spinach.
One medium orange, peeled or sliced

Directions
Combine the tahini, lemon juice, and water in a bowl. Stir in the tuna, olives, feta, and parsley until well combined. Serve the tuna salad over two cups of spinach, with the orange on the side.

Quinoa, Avocado, and Chickpea Salad over Mixed Greens.

Nutrition Facts: 501 Calories, 32g fat, 47g carbs., 12g protein

Prep Time: 20 minutes., Total time: 25 minutes., Servings: Two.

Ingredients
⅔ cup water
⅓ cup quinoa

one-third tsp kosher salt (or coarse salt of choice).
1 clove of garlic, smashed and peeled

2 tablespoons of grated lemon zest.
3 tablespoons of lemon juice.
3 tablespoons of olive oil.
1/4 teaspoon of ground pepper
1 cup of washed, salt-free canned chickpeas
One medium carrot, shredded (1/2 cup)

½ avocado, diced
1 (5-ounce) bag of prewashed mixed greens, such as spring mix or baby kale-spinach blend (8 cups packed).

Directions
Boil water in a small pot. Stir in the quinoa. Reduce the heat to low, cover, and cook for approximately 15 minutes, or until all of the liquid has been absorbed.

Use a fork to fluff and separate the grains; allow to cool for 5 minutes.

Meanwhile, sprinkle salt over the garlic on a chopping board. Mash the garlic with the side of a spoon until it forms a paste.

Scrape into a medium bowl. Whisk in the lemon zest, juice, oil, and pepper. Transfer 3 tablespoons of the dressing to a small dish and set aside.

Toss the chickpeas, carrots, and avocado with the remaining dressing. Allow 5 minutes for the flavors to mingle. Toss gently to coat after adding the quinoa.

Toss the greens in a big dish with the leftover 3 tablespoons of dressing. Divide the greens across two dishes, then top with the quinoa mixture.

Sweet Potato and Cauliflower Rice Bowl

Nutrition Facts: 344 Calories., 18g fat, 39g carbs., 11g protein.

Prep Time: 40 minutes, Total time: 40 minutes., Servings: 4

Ingredients:

1 medium sweet potato, peeled if preferred, and cut 1/4 inch thick.
2 teaspoons extra-virgin olive oil,

2 tablespoons,

2 pinches salt,

1/2 teaspoon ground pepper

1/4 cup orange juice.
2 tablespoons of lime juice.
1/2 cup chopped fresh cilantro, split
3 minced garlic cloves

1/2 teaspoon ground cumin.
½ teaspoon dried oregano.
5 cups cauliflower florets.
1 (15-ounce) can of black beans, rinsed
1 sliced firm ripe avocado and 1/2 cup

pico de gallo.

Directions

Preheat the oven to 400 degrees Fahrenheit.

Toss sweet potatoes in a medium bowl with 2 tablespoons oil, a pinch of salt, and 1/4 teaspoon pepper. Transfer to a baking sheet. Roast until soft, 10 to 14 minutes.

Meanwhile, in a separate bowl, mix the orange juice, lime juice, 1/4 cup cilantro, 1 chopped garlic clove, cumin, oregano, and a sprinkle of salt.

In a food processor, pulse cauliflower florets in two batches until they are roughly the size of rice.In a big pan over medium heat, heat the remaining 2 tablespoons of oil.

Cook until fragrant, approximately 30 seconds, with the remaining 2 garlic cloves.

Cook, stirring, until the cauliflower rice is softened, about 3 to 5 minutes. Remove from heat and add the remaining 1/4 cup cilantro.

To serve, split the cauliflower among four bowls. Top with sweet potatoes, black beans, avocado, and pico de gallo.

Drizzle each serving with the mojo sauce.

Chicken, Avocado, and Quinoa Bowls with Herb Dressing

Nutrition Facts: 753 calories, 50g fat, 43g carbohydrates., 34g protein.

Prep Time: 15 minutes., Cook time: 15 minutes., Total time: 30 minutes., Servings: 4

Ingredients:

Roasted chicken thighs.
Five trimmed, skinless, boneless chicken thighs weighing about 1 1/4 pounds

½ teaspoon ground pepper, ¼ teaspoon salt.

Quinoa
Three cups of low-sodium chicken broth
1 tablespoon of extra virgin olive oil.
¼ teaspoon salt
1 ½ cups quinoa

Italian dressing

¾ cup red wine vinegar.
5 tablespoons water

1 ½ teaspoons sugar

1 tablespoon Dijon mustard.
1 huge clove of garlic.
2 teaspoons dried basil.
2 tablespoons of dried oregano.
½ teaspoon salt.
1/2 teaspoon of ground pepper
1 ¾ cups extra virgin olive oil.

Toppings

1 (15-ounce) can of washed chickpeas
1 sliced avocado

6 thinly sliced radishes

1 cup sprouts or shoots.
1/4 cup toasted seeds or chopped nuts

Directions

To prepare the chicken:

Preheat the oven to 425 degrees Fahrenheit. Place the chicken on a baking sheet. Season with 1/2 teaspoon ground pepper and 1/4 teaspoon salt.

Roast the chicken for 14 to 16 minutes, or until an instant-read thermometer put into the thickest section reads 165 degrees Fahrenheit. Slice four thighs. (Reserve one thigh for another purpose.)

Meanwhile, prepare the quinoa. In a large pot, combine the broth, 1 tablespoon of oil, and 1/4 teaspoon salt. Bring to a simmer over high heat. Stir in the quinoa and bring back to a simmer.

Reduce the heat and let the quinoa absorb all of the liquid and the grains burst, which should take around 15 to 20 minutes.

Remove from heat, cover, and allow it to stand for 5 minutes. (Save two cups for later use.)

To make the dressing, combine vinegar, water, sugar, mustard, garlic, basil, oregano, salt, and pepper in a blender.

Puree till smooth. With the motor running, gradually add the oil and purée until creamy. (Place 1 3/4 cups in a big mason jar and refrigerate for up to a week.).

To arrange the bowls: Divide 3 cups of quinoa into four big, shallow dishes. Add radishes, chickpeas, chicken, sprouts (or shoots), avocado, and seeds (or nuts) on top. Drizzle with 3/4 cup of dressing.

Vegan Grain Bowl

Nutrition Facts: 455 Calories, 25g fat, 51g carbohydrates., 11g protein.

Preparation Time: 30 minutes, Total time: 30 minutes., Servings: 4

Ingredients

1 medium sweet potato, peeled if preferred and chopped into 1-inch slices. Divide 3 tablespoons of extra virgin olive oil,

½ teaspoon of salt,

½ teaspoon of ground pepper.
2 tablespoons tahini.
2 tablespoons of water.
1 tablespoon of lemon juice.
1 small clove of garlic, minced
2 cups of cooked quinoa.
1 15-ounce can of chickpeas, washed
Dice one firm, ripe avocado.

¼ cup minced fresh cilantro or parsley.

Directions

Preheat the oven to 425 degrees Fahrenheit.

In a medium bowl, combine sweet potatoes, 1 tablespoon oil, and 1/4 teaspoon salt and pepper. Transfer to a rimmed baking sheet. Roast, tossing once, until tender, 15 to 18 minutes.

In a separate bowl, mix together the remaining 2 tablespoons oil, tahini, water, lemon juice, garlic, and 1/4 teaspoon salt and pepper.

To serve, divide the quinoa into four bowls. Top with an equal amount of sweet potato, chickpeas, and avocado. Drizzle with tahini sauce. Sprinkle with parsley or cilantro.

Avocado Toast with Burrata.

Nutrition Facts: 439 calories, 28g of fat, 37g of carbohydrates, and 18g of protein.

Prep Time: 5 minutes., Total time: 5 minutes., Servings: One.

Ingredients

1 piece of whole-grain bread (3/4 inch thick).

½ big, ripe avocado, thinly sliced

1 teaspoon of lemon juice.

⅛ teaspoon kosher salt.

1/8 teaspoon ground pepper

1 ½ oz. burrata or fresh mozzarella cheese.

1 teaspoon of freshly chopped fresh basil.

1 teaspoon of minced fresh chives

A pinch of Aleppo pepper.

Directions

Add avocado to the bread. Lemon juice should be drizzled on, and salt and pepper should be added. Sprinkle it with burrata (or mozzarella), basil, chives, and Aleppo pepper.

Stuffed Sweet Potato with Hummus Dressing.

Nutrition Facts: 472 Calories, 7g fat, 85g carbs, 21g protein.

Prep Time: 15 minutes., Total time: 20 minutes., Servings: One.

Ingredients

Scrub 1 big sweet potato and ¾ cup chopped kale.

1 cup rinsed canned black beans and ¼ cup hummus.

2 tablespoons of water.

Directions

Prick the sweet potato all over with a fork. Microwave on high for 7–10 minutes, or until well cooked.

Meanwhile, wash and drain the kale, leaving the water to cling to the leaves. Place in a medium saucepan; cover and cook over medium-high heat, stirring occasionally, until wilted. Add the beans and a tablespoon or two of water if the pot is dry. Continue cooking, uncovered, stirring regularly, until the mixture is boiling hot, about 1 to 2 minutes.

Slice the sweet potato open and top with the kale and bean mixture. In a small bowl, combine the hummus and 2 tablespoons of water. For the right consistency, add more water as needed. Drizzle the hummus dressing over the loaded sweet potatoes.

White Bean and Veggie Salad

Nutrition Facts: 360 Calories, 25g fat, 30g carbs., 10g protein.

Preparation Time: 10 minutes, Total time: 10 minutes., Servings: One.

Ingredients
2 cups mixed salad greens.
¾ cup vegetables of your choosing, such as sliced cucumbers and cherry tomatoes.
⅓ cup canned white beans, washed and strained
½ avocado, diced
1 tablespoon of red wine vinegar.
Two tablespoons of extra-virgin olive oil

¼ teaspoon kosher salt.
Add freshly ground pepper to taste.

Directions
In a medium bowl, combine the greens, vegetables, beans, and avocado. Drizzle with vinegar and oil, then season with salt and pepper. Toss to blend, then transfer to a large platter.

Quick Lentil Salmon Salad.

Nutrition Facts: 341 Calories, 15g fat, 25g carbs., 26g protein.

Cook time: 30 minutes., Total time: 30 minutes., Servings: 4

Ingredients:

¾ cup brown lentils.
½ cup minced red onion

1/4 cup thinly sliced, split
2 garlic cloves, minced
¾ teaspoon salt.
1/4 cup extra virgin olive oil.
3 tablespoons of red wine vinegar.
¾ teaspoon dried thyme.
1/4 teaspoon of ground pepper
1 15-ounce can of salmon, drained
1 cup carrot ribbons.
1 cup sliced celery.
4 lemon wedges to serve.

Directions

Bring some water in a medium saucepan to a boil. Add the lentils and chopped onion, reduce the heat to a brisk simmer, and cook for 11 to 13 minutes, or until just cooked. Drain well.

Meanwhile, crush the garlic and salt together with the side of a chef's knife (or a fork). Transfer to a medium mixing basin and stir in the oil, vinegar, thyme, and pepper.

Remove any skin and/or bones from the salmon and flake it into a large dish.

Toss in the cut onion and carrot, along with 3 tablespoons of the dressing. Add the celery and lentils to the remaining dressing, stirring gently to incorporate.

Divide the lentils amongst four bowls, top with the salmon salad, and serve with lemon wedges.

Roasted Veggie and Tofu Brown Rice Bowl

Nutrition Facts: 454 Calories, 24g fat, 42g carbs., 26g protein.

Prep Time: 5 minutes, Total time: 5 minutes., Servings: One.

Ingredients

½ cup cooked brown rice

1 cup roasted veggies

1 cup of roasted tofu
2 tablespoons of sliced scallions.
2 tablespoons of chopped fresh cilantro.
Two tablespoons. Creamy vegan cashew sauce

Directions

Arrange the rice, vegetables, and tofu in a bowl or 4-cup sealable container. Sprinkle with onions and cilantro. Add cashew sauce over top when ready to serve.

Salmon Salad with Stuffed Avocado

Nutrition Facts: 377 Calories, 24g fat, 20g carbs, 23g protein.

Prep Time: 10 minutes., Total time: 10 minutes., Servings: One.

Ingredients

⅓ cup canned salmon
One spoonful of pesto
1 spoonful of nonfat plain Greek yogurt
2 teaspoons minced shallot.
½ avocado
1 cup baby spinach.
Five tiny wheat crackers.

Directions

Combine salmon, pesto, yogurt, and shallots. Bring some water in a medium saucepan to a boil.

Add cashew sauce over top when ready to serve.

Serve with crackers on the side, and top with avocado and baby spinach.

Kale, Quinoa, and Apple Salad.

Nutrition Facts: 499 Calories, 27g fat, 54g carbs., 13g protein.

Cook Time: 15 minutes., Total time: 15 minutes., Servings: 4

Ingredients

2 teaspoons of cider vinegar.
1 tablespoon of pure maple syrup.
½ teaspoon salt

¼ teaspoon ground pepper

¼ cup extra virgin olive oil.
1 huge bunch of curly kale, stemmed and finely sliced (about 8 cups)
2 medium Honeycrisp or Gala apples, unpeeled and coarsely chopped
1 medium fennel bulb, cored, thinly sliced (3 cups)
2 cups cooked quinoa, room temperature or refrigerated.
1/2 cup roasted slivered almonds (see tip)
⅓ cups dried cherries
1/4 cup crumbled blue cheese.

Directions

Combine vinegar, maple syrup, salt, and pepper in a large basin. Slowly pour in the oil, stirring to mix. With clean hands, massage the kale into the dressing until it is fully coated and somewhat soft, which should take about 3 to 5 minutes.

Toss in the apples, fennel, and quinoa until evenly incorporated. Divide among four dishes, then top with almonds, cherries, and blue cheese.

Tip

To get the finest flavor, roast the nuts before using them in a dish. To toast sliced nuts, set them in a small dry pan and cook over medium-low heat, turning regularly, until fragrant, about 2 to 4 minutes.

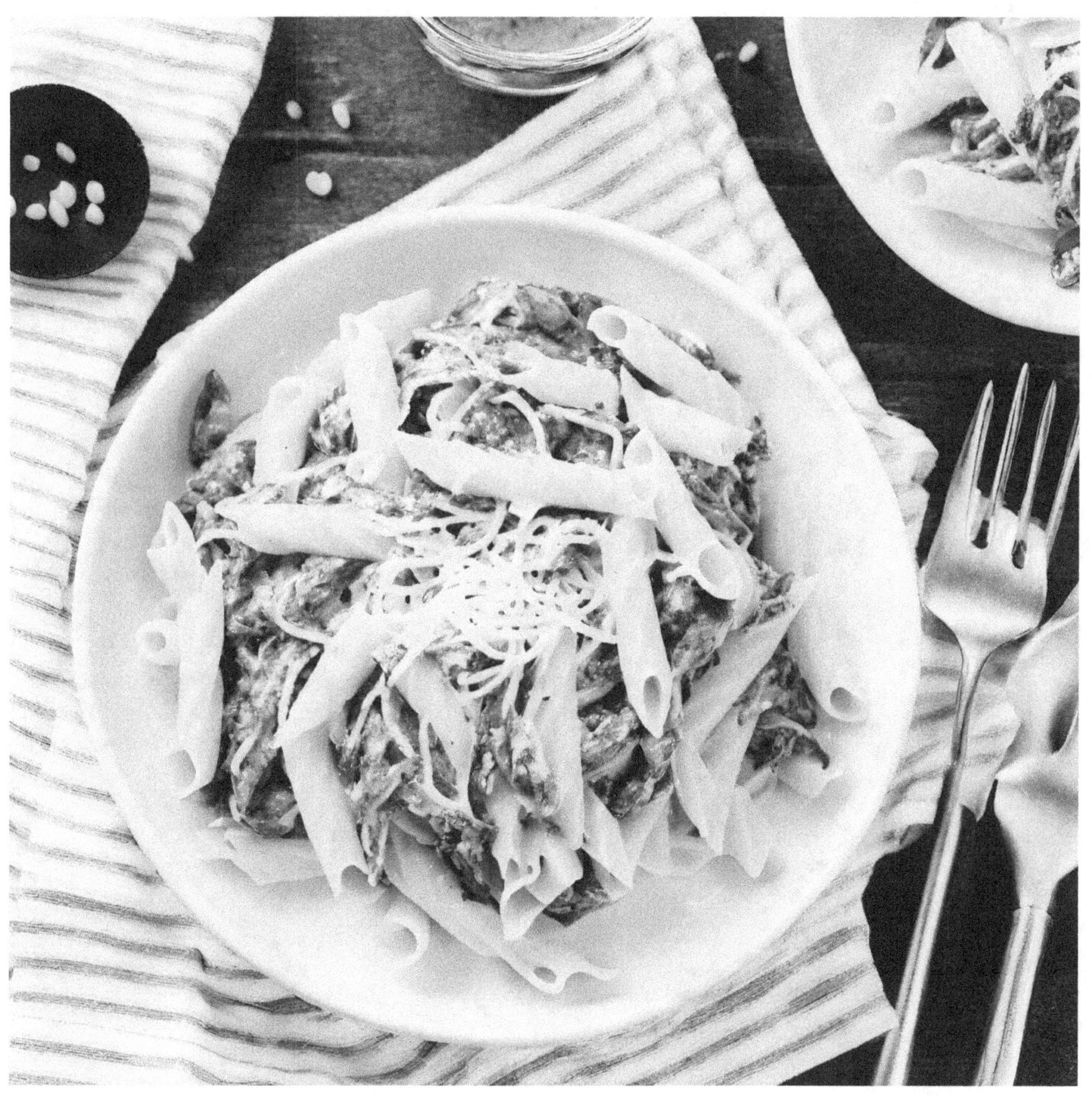

DINNER RECIPES

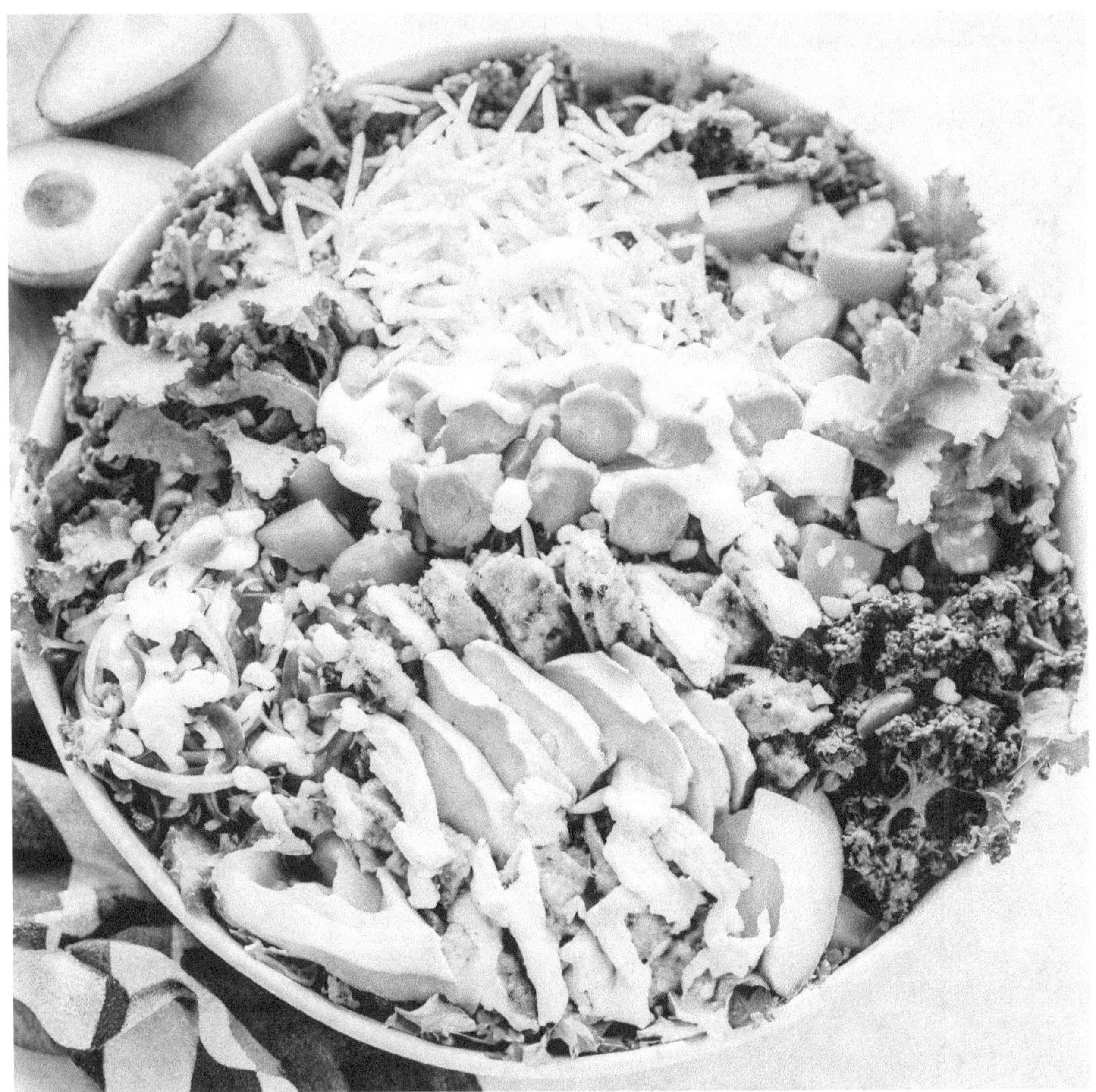

Chicken and Kale Taco Salad with Jalapeño-Avocado Ranch.

Nutrition Facts: 429 calories, 23g fat, 27g carbs, 30g protein.

Prep Time: 25 minutes., Total time: 25 minutes., Serving: 4

Ingredients:

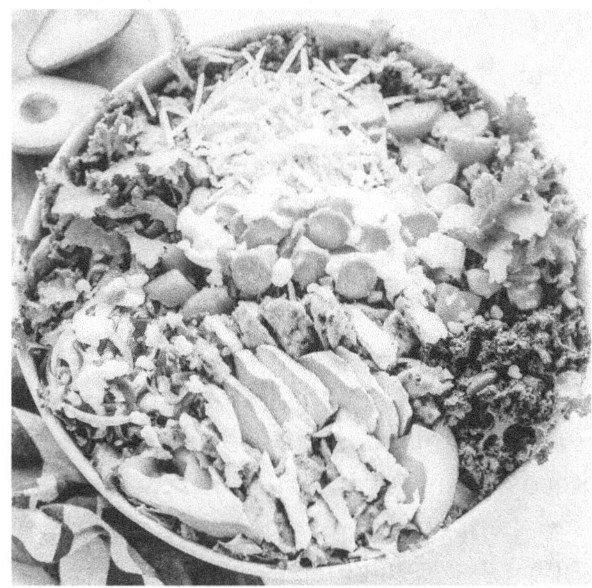

one ripe avocado.
⅓ cup Ranch dressing
2 tablespoons of chopped pickled jalapeños.
1 tablespoon white wine vinegar.
1/4 teaspoon of ground pepper
8 cups shredded kale.

2 cups of shredded cooked chicken breast.
1 1/2 cups of tortilla chips
1 cup canned black beans, rinsed.
1/2 cup chopped mango.
¼ cup shredded cheddar cheese
¼ cup chopped red onions
Lime wedges and crushed red pepper are for serving.

Directions

Mix together avocado, ranch dressing, jalapeños, vinegar, and pepper in a food processor. Pulse until smooth.

In a big bowl, combine the avocado mixture with the kale, chicken, tortilla chips, beans, mango, cheese, and onion. Optional garnishes include lime wedges and crushed red pepper.

Shrimp Bowl Over Brown Rice with Avocado and Tomatoes.

Nutrition Facts: 460 Calories, 22g fat, 40g carbs., 29g protein.

Prep Time: 30 minutes., Total time: 30 minutes., Serving: 4

Ingredients:

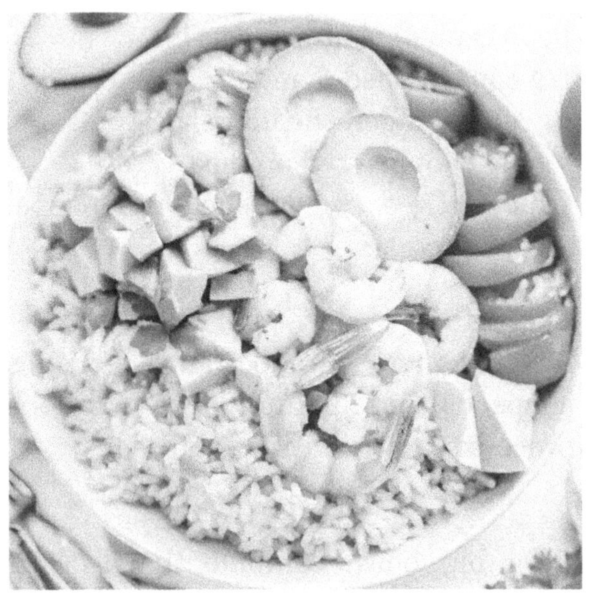

¾ cup finely cut scallion greens.
1/4 cup reduced-sodium tamari
1 ½ teaspoons mirin

1 ½ tablespoons toasted sesame oil (dark).
1 tablespoon of white sesame seeds.
2 teaspoons of grated fresh ginger.
1/2 teaspoon crushed red pepper (optional)

12 ounces cooked shrimp, chopped into half-inch pieces.
2 cups of cooked brown rice.
2 teaspoons of rice vinegar.
2 cups sliced cherry tomatoes.
2 cups chopped avocado.
¼ cup chopped cilantro.
1/4 cup roasted black sesame seeds.

Directions

In a medium bowl, combine the scallion greens, tamari, mirin, oil, white sesame seeds, ginger, and, if desired, crushed red pepper. Set aside 2 tablespoons of sauce in a small dish.

In a medium bowl, combine the shrimp and sauce and gently toss until coated.
In a large bowl, combine the rice and vinegar. Divide among four dishes, then top with 3/4 cup shrimp, 1/2 cup tomatoes and avocado, and 1 tablespoon cilantro and black sesame seeds. Drizzle with the remaining sauce, then serve.

Baked Fish Tacos with Avocado.

Nutrition Facts: 296 Calories., 13g fat, 29g carbs, and 19g protein.

Prep Time: 20 minutes., cook time: 5 minutes., Total time: 25 minutes., Servings: 4

Ingredients

1 tablespoon of avocado oil.
2 tablespoons no salt added Mexican-style seasoning combination.
½ teaspoon salt.
1 pound of flaky white fish filets, such as cod, haddock, or mahi mahi, cut into 8 to 16 pieces
One avocado, sliced into sixteen pieces.
1/2 cup pico de gallo.
8 corn tortillas, warmed

Directions

Preheat the oven to 400 degrees Fahrenheit. Coat a large, rimmed baking sheet with cooking spray.

In a medium bowl, mix together the oil, spice blend, and salt. Add the fish and toss to coat. Transfer to the prepared baking sheet and bake for 10 minutes, or until the fish flakes easily.

To make the tacos, lay 1 or 2 pieces of fish, 2 slices of avocado, and 1 tablespoon pico de gallo in each tortilla.

Quinoa Chickpea Salad with Roasted Red Pepper Hummus Dressing

Nutrition Facts: 379 Calories., 11g fat, 59g carbs., 16g protein.

Prep Time: 10 minutes., Total time: 10 minutes., Servings: 1

Ingredients.

2 tablespoons hummus (original or roasted red pepper taste)
1 tablespoon of lemon juice.
1 tablespoon of chopped roasted red pepper.
2 cups mixed salad greens.
½ cup cooked quinoa.
½ cup washed chickpeas
1 tablespoon of unsalted sunflower

seeds.
1 tablespoon of chopped fresh parsley.
a pinch of salt.
A pinch of ground pepper.

Directions

On a small plate, combine hummus, lemon juice, and red peppers. Thin with water to get the required dressing consistency.

Place the greens, quinoa, and chickpeas in a large bowl. Garnish with sunflower seeds, parsley, salt, and pepper. Serve with the dressing.

Cauliflower Rice Bowls with Grilled Chicken

Nutrition Facts: 411 Calories, 28g fat, 10g carbs., 29g protein.

Prep Time: 30 minutes., Total time: 30 minutes., Servings: 4

Ingredients:

6 tablespoons and 1 teaspoon extra virgin olive oil, divided
4 cups cauliflower rice (see tip)
⅓ cup diced red onion
¾ teaspoon salt, divided.
1/2 cup chopped fresh dill, divided.
1 pound of boneless, skinless chicken breasts.
1/2 teaspoon ground pepper, divided
3 tablespoons of lemon juice.
1 teaspoon of dried oregano.
1 cup halved cherry tomatoes.
1 cup of diced cucumber.
2 tablespoons chopped Kalamata olives.
2 tablespoons of crumbled feta cheese.
Four wedges. Lemon wedges for serving.

Directions

Preheat the grill to medium.
Heat 2 tablespoons of oil in a large pan over medium-high heat. Combine the cauliflower, onion, and 1/4 teaspoon salt. Cook, stirring occasionally, until the cauliflower softens, about 5 minutes. Remove from heat and add 1/4 cup dill.

Meanwhile, spread 1 teaspoon of oil all over the chicken. Add 1/4 teaspoon each of salt and pepper for seasoning. Grill, flipping once, until an instant-read thermometer placed into the thickest portion of the breast registers 165 degrees Fahrenheit, about 15 minutes total. Cut crosswise.

Meanwhile, in a separate dish, combine the remaining 4 tablespoons oil, lemon juice, oregano, and 1/4 teaspoon salt and pepper.

Divide the cauliflower rice into four dishes. Top with chicken, tomatoes, cucumber, olives, and feta. Sprinkle with the remaining 1/4 cup of dill. Drizzle with vinaigrette. Serve with lemon slices, if preferred.

Tip
Look for prepared cauliflower rice (or crumbled cauliflower) at different grocery stores along with other cooked vegetables. To create your own, put cauliflower florets in a food processor and pulse until they are broken down into rice-sized grains. A 2-pound head of cauliflower provides around 4 cups of cauliflower rice.

Sheet Pan Chili Lime Salmon with Potatoes and Peppers

Nutrition Facts: 405 Calories, 17g fat, 26g carbohydrates., 35g protein.

Prep Time: 25 minutes., Total time: 25 minutes., Servings: 4

Ingredients
1 pound Yukon Gold potatoes, chopped into 3/4-inch chunks
2 tablespoons extra virgin olive oil,

¾ teaspoon salt

¼ teaspoon ground pepper.
2 teaspoons of chili powder.
1 teaspoon ground cumin.
½ teaspoon garlic powder.
One lime, zested and quartered
slice 2 medium bell peppers of any color

1 ¼ pounds of center-cut salmon filet, peeled if preferred and chopped into 4 parts.

Directions
Preheat the oven to 425 degrees Fahrenheit. Coat a large, rimmed baking sheet with cooking spray.

In a larger bowl, toss potatoes with 1 tablespoon oil, 1/4 teaspoon salt, and pepper. Transfer to the preheated pan and roast for 15 minutes.

Meanwhile, in a separate bowl, add the chili powder, cumin, garlic powder, lime zest, and remaining 1/2 teaspoon salt. In a medium bowl, combine the bell peppers, remaining 1 tablespoon oil, and 1/2 tablespoon spice mixture; toss to coat. Coat the salmon with the remaining spice mix.

Remove the pan from the oven after 15 minutes. Stir in the peppers until well combined. Roast for five minutes.

Remove from the oven, transfer some of the veggies, and add the salmon to the pan. Roast the fish for 6 to 8 minutes, or until just cooked through. Serve with lime wedges.

Creamy Spinach Pasta

Nutrition Facts: 395 Calories, 16g fat, 50g carbs., 23g protein.

Prep Time: 15 minutes, Total time: 15 minutes., Servings: 4

Ingredients

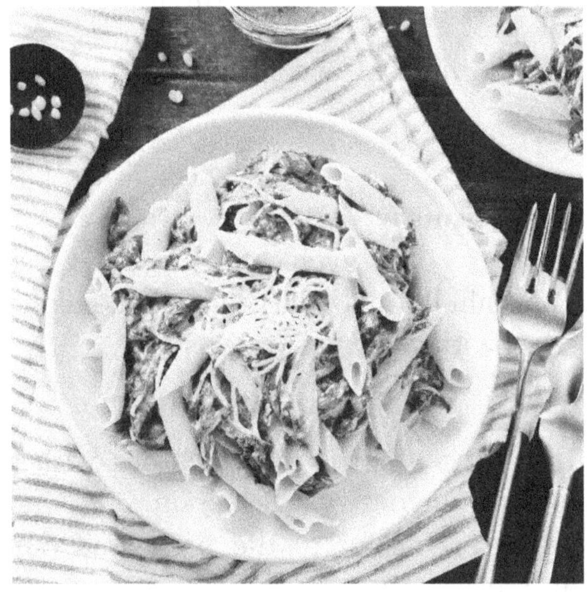

12 ounces of uncooked tube-shaped chickpea pasta (about 3 1/2 cups) (like Banza
1 garlic clove, finely sliced (approximately 1 tsp.)
2 tablespoons of finely sliced shallot
3 ¼ oz. mascarpone cheese
4 ounces of fresh baby spinach.

1 teaspoon of kosher salt.
½ teaspoon black pepper.
1 teaspoon of lemon zest (from one lemon)
One pinch of crushed red pepper

Directions

Cook the pasta according to the package guidelines, omitting salt. Reserve 1 cup of the cooking water and drain. In a large bowl, combine pasta, garlic, shallot, mascarpone, spinach, salt, pepper, and 1/2 cup of the saved cooking liquid.

Stir for 1 1/2 minutes, or until the cheese has melted and the mixture is well blended. Add more cooking liquid as needed to loosen the sauce. Divide the spaghetti among four bowls. Season with lemon zest and, if preferred, crushed red pepper. Serve immediately.

Lemon Garlic Pasta with Salmon

Nutrition Facts: 473 Calories, 23g fat, 49g carbs., 20g protein.

Prep Time: 15 minutes., Total time: 15 minutes., Servings: 4

Ingredients
8 ounces of whole wheat pasta

5 tablespoons of extra virgin olive oil.
5 cloves of garlic, chopped
1 teaspoon of anchovy paste.
¼ teaspoon crushed red pepper.
Zest and juice of one lemon
1 1/2 cups flakes of cooked salmon
3 tablespoons chopped fresh parsley

 ¼ teaspoon salt.
2 tablespoons toasted whole-wheat breadcrumbs.

Directions
Cook pasta according to the package guidelines. Save half a cup of the cooking water and drain.

In a large pan, combine the oil, garlic, anchovy paste, crushed red pepper, lemon zest, and juice. Heat over medium-high heat for 3 minutes, or until sizzling.

Add the conserved water, pasta, fish, parsley, and salt. Cook, tossing, for approximately 2 minutes, or until the sauce has coated the pasta. Serve, topped with breadcrumbs.

Crispy Fish Taco Bowls.

Nutrition Facts: 478 Calories., 25g fat, 42g carbs., 20g protein.

Prep Time: 20 minutes., Total time: 20 minutes., Servings: 4

Ingredients
Cut 1 pound of white fish, such as cod, into 2-inch pieces.
1/2 cup mayonnaise, split

¾ cup panko breadcrumbs
1/4 cup sour cream.
2 tablespoons of adobo sauce made from chipotle peppers

2 tablespoons of lime juice.
A pinch of salt and 1/4 teaspoon of ground pepper, divided.
2 cups of cooked brown rice.
2 cups shredded cabbage.
1 cup finely sliced radishes.
Fresh cilantro for garnish.

Directions

Preheat the oven to 475 degrees Fahrenheit. Arrange a wire rack onto a baking sheet with a rim and mist with cooking spray. Coat the fish with 1/4 cup of mayonnaise. Place the panko in a shallow dish and coat the fish in it. Transfer to the rack in the pan.

Bake the fish until crispy and cooked through, which should take 8 to 12 minutes, depending on thickness. Meanwhile, combine the remaining 1/4 cup mayonnaise, sour cream, adobo sauce, lime juice, and a sprinkle of salt in a small dish.

Season the fish with the remaining 1/4 teaspoon of salt and pepper. Divide the rice into four bowls and top with the fish, cabbage, radishes, sauce, and cilantro, if preferred.

Salmon-Stuffed Avocados

Nutrition Facts: 293 Calories., 20g fat, 11g carbohydrates., 23g protein.

Prep Time: 15 minutes., Total time: 15 minutes.,four servings

Ingredients:.

1/2 cup nonfat plain Greek yogurt
1/2 cup chopped celery.
2 tablespoons of chopped fresh parsley.
1 tablespoon of lime juice.
2 tsp. mayonnaise
1 teaspoon Dijon mustard.
⅛ teaspoon salt.
1/8 teaspoon ground pepper
Two (5-ounce) cans of salmon, drained, flakes, skin, and bones removed.
Two avocados.
Chopped chives as garnish

Directions

In a medium bowl, combine the yogurt, celery, parsley, lime juice, mayonnaise, mustard, salt, and pepper. Mix thoroughly. Add the fish and stir thoroughly.

Halve avocados lengthwise and remove the pits. Scoop approximately 1 tablespoon of flesh from each avocado half into a small dish. Mash the scooped-out avocado flesh with a fork and add it to the salmon mixture.

Fill each avocado half with about 1/4 cup of the salmon mixture and mound it on top. Garnish with chives, if desired.

Vegan Coconut Chickpea Curry

Nutrition Facts: 471 calories, 18g fat, 66g carbs., 11g protein.

Preparation Time: 20 minutes, Total time: 20 minutes., Servings: 4

Ingredients
2 teaspoons of avocado or canola oil
1 cup minced onion, 1 cup diced bell pepper.
One medium zucchini, halved and sliced
One fifteen-ounce can (drained and rinsed) of chickpeas

1 ½ cups coconut curry simmer sauce
1/2 cup veggie broth.
4 cups baby spinach.
2 cups of precooked brown rice, prepared according to the package directions.

Directions
In a large skillet, heat the oil over medium-high heat. Cook, turning often, until the onion, pepper, and zucchini begin to brown, about 5 to 6 minutes.

Add chickpeas, simmer sauce, and broth, and bring to a simmer while stirring. Reduce the heat to medium-low and cook until the veggies are soft, about 4 to 6 minutes. Stir in the spinach right before serving. Serve over rice.

Salmon Tacos with Pineapple Salsa

Nutrition Facts: 320 Calories, 11g fat, 30g carbs., 26g protein.

Prep Time: 20 minutes., Total time: 20 minutes., Servings: 4

Ingredients

1 (1 pound) salmon filet.
1 teaspoon of chili powder.
¾ teaspoon salt

One tablespoon of extra virgin olive oil and one teaspoon of it, divided.

1 package of coleslaw mix (9 ounces, 5 cups)
Juice half a lime and reheat 8 (6-inch) corn tortillas
¾ cup bought pineapple salsa

Chopped fresh cilantro for garnish.
Hot Sauce for Serving

Directions

Arrange the oven rack in the upper part of the oven, so the salmon is 2 to 3 inches below the heat source. Preheat the broiler too high.

Line a baking pan with foil. Place the skin side down of the fish onto the foil.

Broil, moving the pan from front to back once, until the salmon begins to brown, is opaque on the sides, and the thinner areas of the filet sizzle, 5 to 8 minutes, depending on thickness.

Season the fish with chili powder and 1/4 teaspoon salt. To moisten the spices, drizzle with 1 teaspoon of oil and use a heatproof brush. Return to the oven and continue broiling until the salmon flakes and the spices are browned, about 1 to 2 minutes longer.

Meanwhile, combine the coleslaw mix with the lime juice, remaining 1 tablespoon oil, and 1/2 teaspoon salt. Flake the fish and discard the skin. Divide the salmon between the tortillas and top with salsa. Serve with coleslaw, and if preferred, sprinkle with cilantro and spicy sauce.

Skillet Lemon Chicken with Spinach

Nutrition Facts: 317 Calories, 16g fat, 11g carbohydrates., 26g protein.

Cook Time: 25 minutes., Total time: 25 minutes., Servings: 4

Ingredients

2 tablespoons extra virgin olive oil
1 pound boneless, skinless chicken thighs, trimmed and chopped into bite-sized pieces.
1 cup of chopped red bell pepper.
½ teaspoon salt.
1/2 teaspoon of ground pepper
4 garlic cloves, minced
1/2 cup dry white wine.
1 teaspoon cornstarch.
1 medium lemon, zested and squeezed
10 cups of thinly packed baby spinach.
8 tsp. grated Parmesan cheese

Directions

In a large skillet, heat the oil over medium-high heat. Cook, tossing occasionally, until the chicken is just cooked through, about 7 to 9 minutes. Stir in the garlic and simmer for about a minute, or until fragrant.

In a measuring cup, whisk together the wine and cornstarch. Add to the pan, along with the lemon juice and zest, and swirl to coat. Bring to a boil. Cook, stirring, until the spinach is wilted, approximately 2 minutes. Serve sprinkled with Parmesan cheese.

Salmon with Lemon-Herb Orzo and Broccoli.

Nutrition Facts: 425 Calories., 17g fat, 32g carbs., 35g protein.

Cook Time: 25 minutes., Total time: 25 minutes., Servings: 4

Ingredients

1 cup orzo (ideally whole-wheat)
2 cups chopped broccoli (about 1/2 head)
Divide 3 tablespoons of extra virgin olive oil and 1 ¼ pounds of skin-on salmon filet into 4 parts. Pat dry.
½ teaspoon salt

½ teaspoon ground pepper, divided
4 tablespoons of chopped fresh herbs, such as tarragon, chives, and/or parsley.
2 tbsp. lemon zest
1 tablespoon of lemon juice.

Directions

In a large saucepan, bring two quarts of water to a boil. Cook the orzo according to the package guidelines, adding the broccoli for the final minute. Drain and rinse in cool water.

Meanwhile, heat 1 1/2 teaspoons of oil in a large nonstick pan over medium-high heat. Season the fish with 1/4 teaspoon salt and pepper. Cook, skin side up, until golden brown, 3 to 5 minutes. Flip and cook until the meat is opaque, which should take 3 to 5 minutes, depending on thickness.

In a medium bowl, combine 2 tablespoons of oil, herbs, lemon zest, lemon juice, and the remaining 1/4 teaspoon each of salt and pepper. Stir in the orzo and broccoli until evenly incorporated.

Serve the orzo mixture with the fish, drizzled with the remaining 1 1/2 tablespoons of oil.

Quinoa Chili with Sweet Potatoes

Nutrition Facts: 346 Calories, 6g fat, 63g carbs., 12g protein

Cook Time: 15 minutes., Total time: 30 minutes., Servings: 5

Ingredients:

1 tablespoon extra virgin olive oil.
2 (12 ounces) sweet potatoes, peeled and sliced into half-inch chunks
One medium yellow onion, chopped
2 poblano peppers, diced
Four big cloves of garlic, chopped
1 tablespoon of chili powder.
2 tablespoons ground cumin
4 cups of unsalted vegetable broth.
One (10-ounce) can of no-salted diced tomatoes with green chilies
1 (4-ounce) can of chopped green chiles
Two cups of water, divided
1 cup uncooked white or multicolored quinoa.
1 (15-ounce) can of no-salted pinto beans, rinsed
½ teaspoon salt.
sliced jalapeño peppers, yogurt, and cilantro.

Directions

Heat the oil in a big saucepan over medium-high heat. Cook, tossing occasionally, until the sweet potatoes are slightly softened and faintly browned, about 6 to 7 minutes. Cook, stirring periodically, for 3 minutes, or until the onion and poblanos are somewhat softened.

Cook, stirring regularly, until the garlic, chili powder, and cumin are fragrant, approximately 30 seconds. Combine broth, tomatoes, green chilies, and 1 cup water. Cover, turn the heat up to high, and bring to a boil.

Stir in the quinoa, beans, and salt. Reduce the heat to medium, cover, and simmer, stirring periodically, until the quinoa is cooked, about 15 minutes. Add the remaining 1 cup of water during the final 3 minutes of cooking. Garnish with jalapeño slices, yogurt, and cilantro as desired.

Creamy Salmon Pasta with Sundried Tomatoes

Nutrition Facts: 458 Calories, 14g fat, 60g carbs., 27g protein.

Cook Time: 20 minutes., Total time: 25 minutes., Servings: 6.

Ingredients

1 pound of whole wheat rigatoni.

Chop ¼ cup oil-packed sun-dried tomatoes and add 2 tablespoons of oil from the container (or 2 tablespoons olive oil), divided.

One big shallot, coarsely chopped

2 garlic cloves, minced

½ cup half-and-half, 1/2 cup unsalted chicken, or veggie broth.

1 teaspoon salt.

1 ½ cups of fresh basil leaves, loosely packed.

12 oz. cooked or canned salmon, flaked into 1-inch pieces.

2 teaspoons of lemon juice.

1/4 cup chopped fresh flat-leaf parsley.

Directions

Bring a kettle of water to a boil. Cook pasta according to package directions until 1 minute before al dente; drain and set aside.

Meanwhile, warm sun-dried tomato oil (or olive oil) in a large nonstick pan over medium-high heat. Cook, stirring often, until the shallot is transparent, which should take around 1 minute. Combine sun-dried tomatoes, half-and-half, broth, and salt. Bring to a simmer on medium-high heat.

Reduce the heat to medium and simmer, stirring periodically, for 5 to 7 minutes, or until slightly thickened and reduced.

Combine the spaghetti with the tomato mixture in the pan.

Cook for 2 minutes over medium heat, tossing regularly to ensure that the pasta is uniformly coated. Stir in the basil.

Remove from heat. Fold in the fish and lemon juice gently. Sprinkle with parsley, and serve.

One-Pot Chicken and Broccoli Pasta

Nutrition Facts: 530 Calories., 18g fat, 52g carbs., 44g protein.

Cook Time: 20 minutes, Total time: 20 minutes., Servings: 4

Ingredients
Combine 2 cups of unsalted chicken broth and 2 cups of water.
8 ounces of whole grain, tiny shell pasta.
2 tablespoons extra virgin olive oil
1 ½ teaspoons Worcestershire sauce.
1 tablespoon of unsalted tomato paste.
3 garlic cloves, minced
½ teaspoon ground pepper, ¼ teaspoon salt.
12 ounces of broccoli florets, chopped into bite-sized pieces
2 cups of shredded cooked chicken breast.
¾ cup plain Greek yogurt with whole milk
¾ cup grated Parmesan cheese, split
2 tablespoons of chopped fresh dill.

Directions
In a large saucepan or high-sided skillet, combine the broth, water, pasta, oil, Worcestershire sauce, tomato paste, garlic, pepper, and salt. Over high heat, bring to a boil, stirring occasionally.

Cook, tossing frequently to keep the pasta from sticking, until al dente, the broccoli is soft, and the sauce is creamy, about 7 to 8 minutes.

Remove from heat and mix in the chicken, yogurt, Parmesan, and dill.

Kale and Quinoa Salad with Lemon Dressing.

Nutrition Facts : 400 Calories, 23g fat, 37g carbs., 14g protein.

Cook Time: 25 minutes., Total time: 25 minutes., Servings: 6.

Ingredients:

One bunch of chopped and stemmed lacinato kale.

Six tablespoons of extra-virgin olive oil
3 tablespoons of lemon juice.
2 teaspoons chopped shallots
1 teaspoon honey.
½ teaspoon salt, ¼ teaspoon ground pepper.
2 cups grape or cherry tomatoes, halved
2 cups of cooked quinoa.
One English cucumber, thinly sliced
1 medium-sliced red bell pepper, 1 medium-sliced yellow bell pepper

1 (15-ounce) can of rinsed unsalted chickpeas

¾ cup crumbled feta cheese

½ cup toasted sliced almonds.

Directions
Place the kale in a large serving basin. In a small bowl, whisk together the oil, lemon juice, shallot, honey, salt, and pepper.

Add two to three tablespoons of the dressing to the kale and massage it gently for one to two minutes, or until the kale begins to wilt slightly.

Top the kale with tomatoes, quinoa, cucumbers, peppers, chickpeas, feta, and almonds. Drizzle with the remaining dressing and mix before serving.

One-Pot Garlic Shrimp with Spinach

Nutrition Facts: 226 Calories, 12g fat, 6g carbs, 26g protein.

Cook Time: 25 minutes., Total time: 25 minutes., Servings: 4

Ingredients

3 tablespoons of extra virgin olive oil, divided.
6 medium cloves of garlic, cut and split.
1/4 cup salt (plus 1/8 teaspoon), mixed into 1 pound of spinach.

1 tablespoon of lemon juice.
1 pound peeled and deveined shrimp (21–30 count)

¼ teaspoon crushed red pepper.
1 tablespoon of freshly chopped fresh parsley.
1 ½ teaspoon lemon zest.

Directions

In a big saucepan, heat 1 tablespoon of oil over medium heat. Add half of the garlic and sauté for 1 to 2 minutes, until it begins to brown. Toss in spinach and 1/4 teaspoon salt until well coated.

Simmer for 3 to 5 minutes, stirring once or twice, or until mostly wilted. After taking off the heat, stir in the lemon juice. Transfer to a bowl to keep warm. Increase the heat to medium-high and add the remaining 2 tablespoons of oil to the saucepan.

Cook until the remaining garlic begins to brown, about 1 to 2 minutes. Add the shrimp, crushed red pepper, and the remaining 1/8 teaspoon salt; simmer, tossing, until the shrimp are just cooked through, 3 to 5 minutes longer. Sprinkle the shrimp with lemon zest and parsley before serving over spinach.

This simple and flavorful dish may be served over spaghetti, orzo, or brown rice, or on its own with a side of crusty bread to soak up any remaining sauce.

To liven things up, top it with Parmesan cheese or chopped fresh herbs like basil or chives in addition to parsley, as well as more lemon juice and zest for a tangy kick.

Quinoa with Chickpeas Roasted Red pepper Sauce

Nutrition Facts: 479 Calories, 25g fat, 50g carbs., 13g protein.

Prep Time: 20 minutes., Total time: 20 minutes., Servings: 4

Ingredients

1 (7-ounce) container of rinsed roasted red peppers

¼ cup of slivered almonds.
4 tablespoons of extra virgin olive oil, split
1 small clove of garlic, minced
1 teaspoon of paprika.
1/2 teaspoon ground cumin
¼ teaspoon of crushed red pepper (optional)
Add 2 cups cooked quinoa,

¼ cup chopped Kalamata olives

¼ cup finely chopped red onion.
1 (15-ounce) can of washed chickpeas
1 cup of chopped cucumber.
1/4 cup crumbled feta cheese.
2 tablespoons of freshly chopped fresh parsley.

Directions

Place the almonds, garlic, paprika, cumin, crushed red pepper (if using), peppers, and two tablespoons of oil in a small food processor. Puree until somewhat smooth.

In a medium bowl, combine the quinoa, olives, red onion, and remaining 2 tablespoons of oil.

To serve, divide the quinoa mixture among four bowls and top with equal parts chickpeas, cucumber, and red pepper sauce. Sprinkle with feta and parsley.

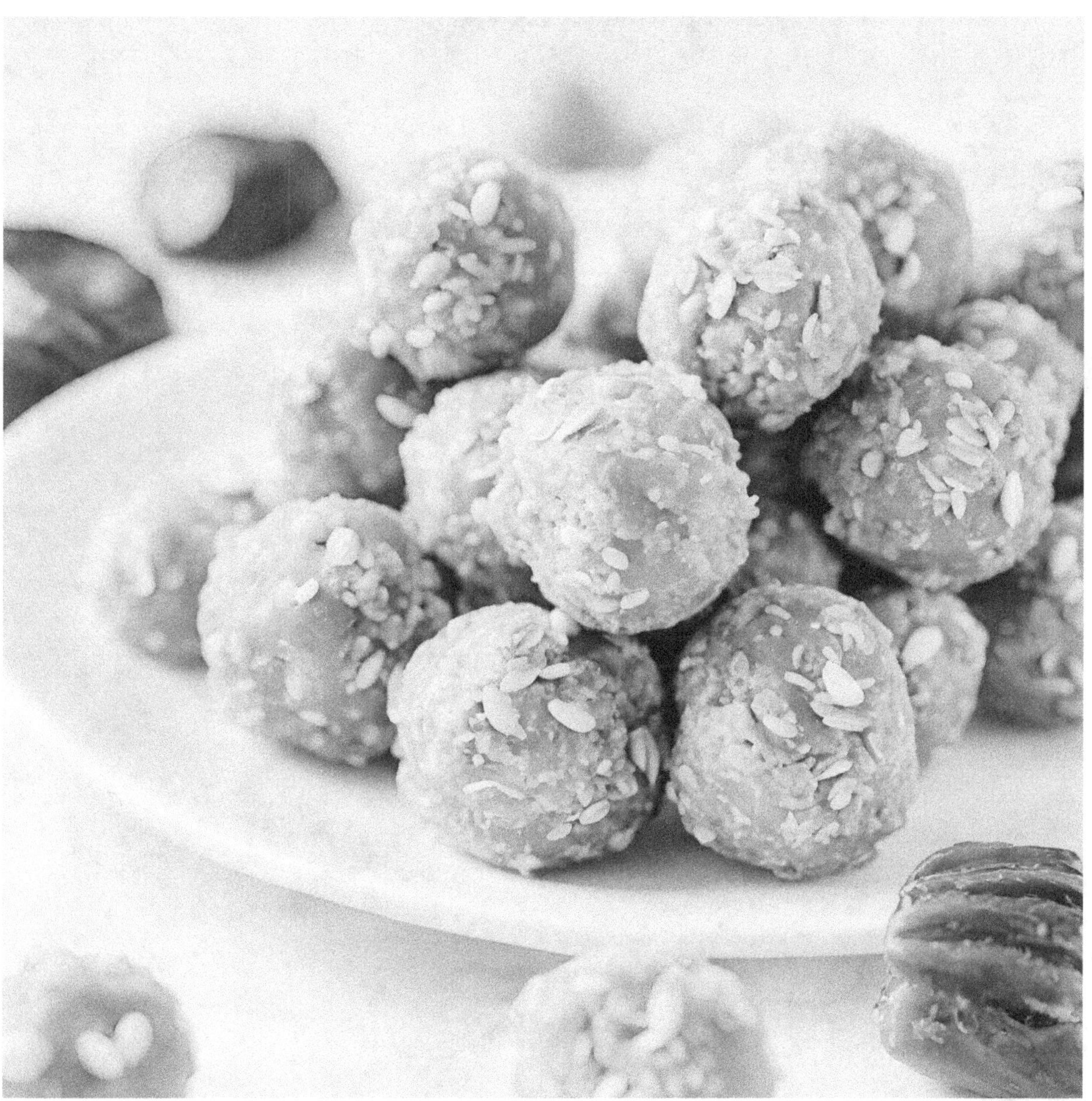

APPETIZER AND SNACKS

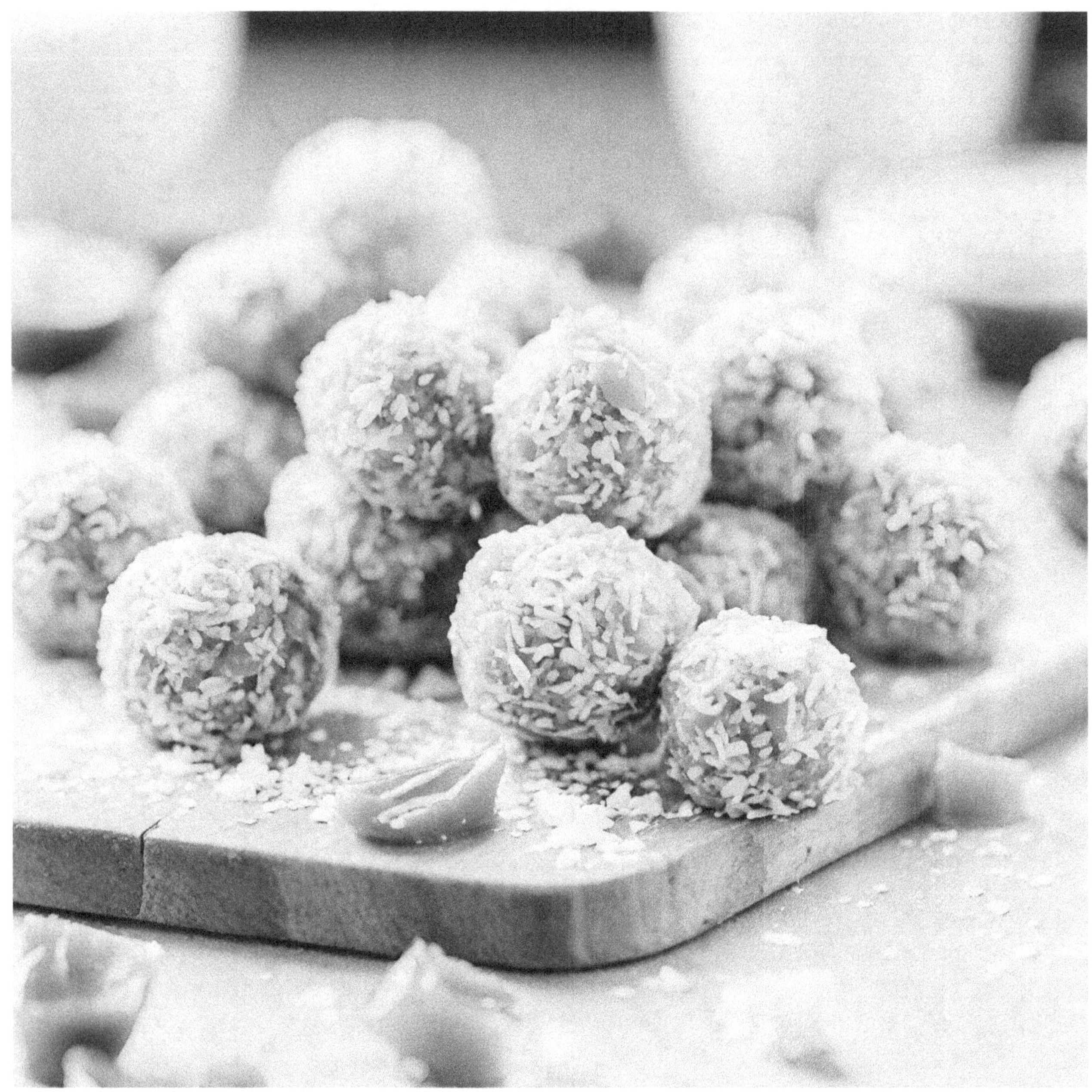

Peanut Butter-Date Energy Balls

Nutrition Facts: 75 Calories., 3g fat, 10g carbohydrates., 2g protein.

Prep Time: 25 minutes, Total time: 25 minutes., Servings: 32.

Ingredients:

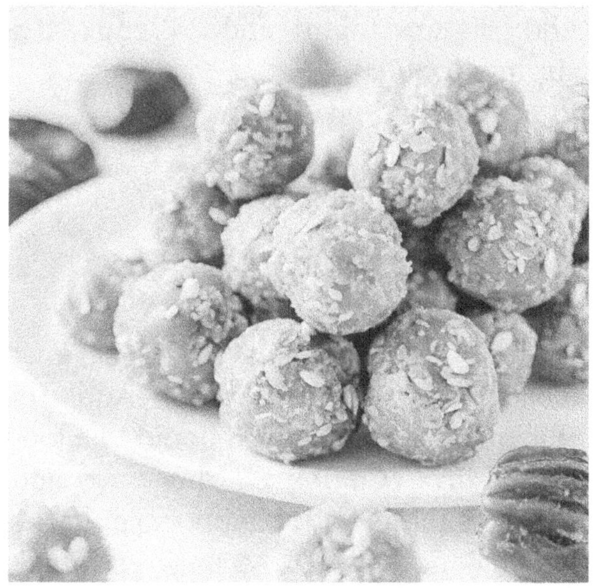

2 ¼ cups roughly chopped pitted dates.
½ cup of puffed amaranth cereal or brown rice

¾ cup creamy peanut butter
3 tablespoons ground flaxseed.
a pinch of salt.

Directions

Blend dates, cereal, peanut butter, flaxseed, and salt in a food processor. Pulse 10 to 20 times until finely chopped, then process for approximately 1 minute, scraping down the sides as needed, until the mixture is crumbly but holds together when pushed.

Squeeze roughly 1 tablespoon of the mixture tightly between your palms and roll into a ball. Place it in a storage container. Repeat with the remaining mixture.

Avocado Hummus

Nutrition Facts: 156 Calories, 12g fat, 10g carbs., 3g protein.

Preparation time: 10 minutes., Total time: 10 minutes., Servings: 10

Ingredients:

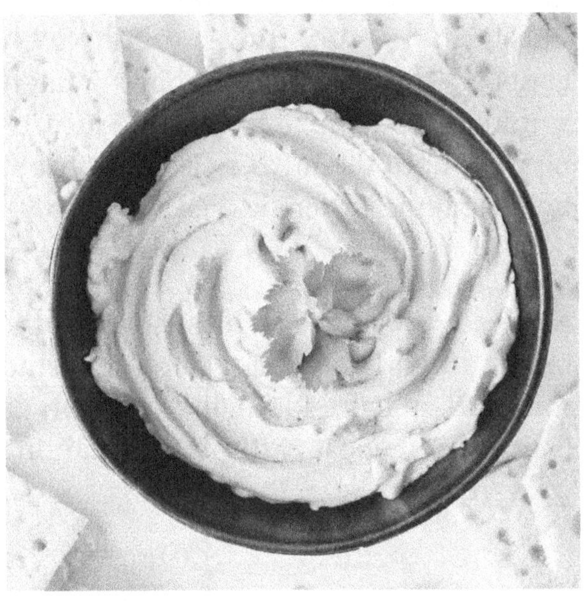

1 (15 oz.) can of chickpeas with salt added
1 ripe avocado, halved and pitted; 1 cup fresh cilantro leaves.
Add ¼ cup tahini and ¼ cup extra virgin olive oil.
¼ cup lemon juice
1 clove of garlic.
1 teaspoon ground cumin.
½ teaspoon salt.

Directions

Drain the chickpeas and save 2 tablespoons of the liquid. Add the chickpeas and conserved liquid to a food processor. Combine the avocado, cilantro, tahini, oil, lemon juice, garlic, cumin, and salt. Puree until extremely smooth. Serve with vegetables, pita chips, or crudités.

Peanut Butter Energy Balls.

Nutrition Facts: 174 Calories, 9g fat, 18g carbohydrates., 4g protein.

Prep Time: 20 minutes., Total time: 20 minutes., Total servings: 17.

Ingredients

2 cups of rolled oats (see Tip).
One cup of natural peanut butter, or another type of nut butter

½ cup honey
1/4 cup micro-chocolate chips.
1/4 cup unsweetened shredded coconut.

Directions

In a medium bowl, combine oats, peanut butter (or other nut butter), honey, chocolate chips, and coconut. Stir thoroughly. Roll the mixture into 1-tablespoon-sized balls.

Tip

People with celiac disease or gluten sensitivity should use "gluten-free" oats, as they are frequently cross-contaminated with wheat and barley.

Garlic Hummus.

Nutrition Facts: 155 Calories., 12g fat, 10g carbs., 4g protein.

Cook Time: 10 minutes., Total time: 10 minutes., Servings: 8

Ingredients:

1 (15 oz.) can chickpeas with salt

¼ cup tahini

¼ cup extra virgin olive oil

¼ cup lemon juice.
1 clove of garlic.
1 teaspoon ground cumin.
½ teaspoon chili powder.
½ teaspoon salt.

Directions

Drain the chickpeas and save 1/4 cup of the liquid. Add the chickpeas and conserved liquid to a food processor.

Combine the tahini, oil, lemon juice, garlic, cumin, chili powder, and salt. Puree for 2-3 minutes, or until extremely smooth.

Peanut Butter Blueberry Energy Balls.

Nutrition Facts: 183 Calories, 9g fat, 20g carbs., 5g protein.

Cook Time: 20 minutes., Total time: 20 minutes., Total servings: 17.

Ingredients

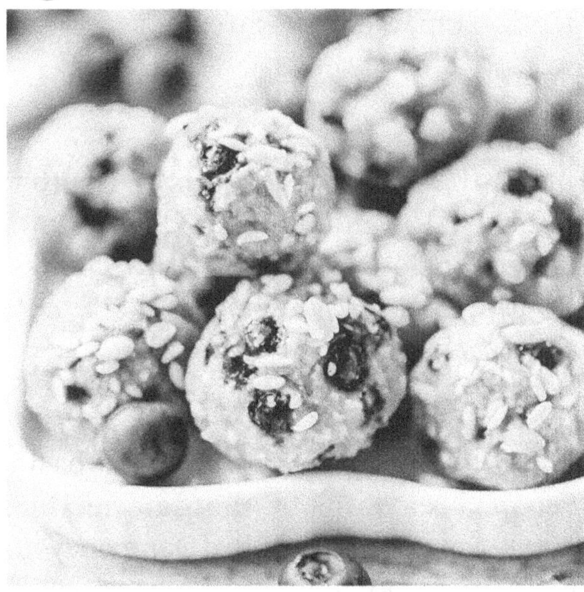

2 cups of rolled oats (see Tip).
One cup of natural peanut butter, or another type of nut butter

½ cup honey and ¼ cup small chocolate chips.
¼ cup dried blueberries

Directions

In a medium bowl, combine oats, peanut butter (or other nut butter), honey, chocolate chips, and blueberries. Stir thoroughly.

Roll the mixture into 1-tablespoon-sized balls. Refrigerate in an airtight container for up to 5 days, or freeze for up to 3 months.

Tip

People with celiac disease or gluten sensitivity should use "gluten-free" oats, as they are frequently cross-contaminated with wheat and barley.

Salted Coconut and Caramel Energy Balls

Nutrition Facts: 100 Calories, 5g fat, 14g carbohydrates, and 2g protein.

Prep Time: 30 minutes., Total time: 30 minutes., Servings: 36.

Ingredients

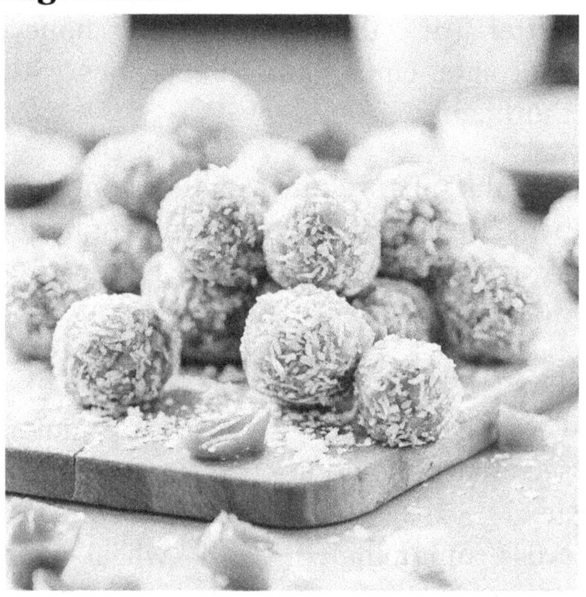

Four dozen pitted dates (about three cups)
¾ cup creamy sunflower seed butter
6 tablespoons of warm water.
1 ½ teaspoon kosher salt.
1 ¼ teaspoon vanilla extract.
2 cups of rolled oats (see Tip).
6 tablespoons of roughly chopped, toasted pecans

1/2 cup unsweetened shredded coconut.

Directions
Blend the dates, sunflower seed butter, water, salt, and vanilla. Blend until largely smooth, with a few tiny chunks. Transfer to a medium bowl. Add the oats and pecans, stirring thoroughly.

Place the coconuts in a small basin. Scoop a spoonful of the date mixture and form it into a ball. (Dampen your hands to avoid sticking.) Roll the ball in coconut to coat. Repeat with the remaining mixture.

Tip: People with celiac disease or gluten sensitivity should use "gluten-free" oats, as they are frequently cross-contaminated with wheat and barley.

Mango-Date Energy Bites.

Nutrition Facts: 73 Calories., 3g fat, 11g carbohydrates., 1g protein.

Cook time: 15 minutes., Total time: 15 minutes., Servings: 20.

Ingredients
Two cups of pitted whole dates
1 cup raw cashews.
1 cup dried mango or another dry fruit.
¼ teaspoon salt

Directions
In a food processor, combine dates, cashews, mango (or other fruit), and salt until finely minced. Form into roughly 20 balls with 2 tablespoons each.

Savory Date and Pistachio Bites

Nutrition Facts: 68 Calories., 2g fat, 13g carbs., 1g protein.

Prep Time: 10 minutes., Total time: 10 minutes., Servings: 32.

Ingredients:

2 cups of pitted whole dates.
1 cup raw, unsalted, shelled pistachios
1 cup golden raisins.
1 teaspoon of powdered fennel seeds.
1/4 teaspoon of ground pepper

Directions
Mix dates, pistachios, raisins, fennel, and pepper in a food processor. Process until finely chopped. Form into approximately 32 balls, each containing about 1 tablespoon.

Peanut Butter and Oat Energy Balls

Nutrition Facts: 73 Calories., 3g fat, 10g carbohydrates., 2g protein.

Prep Time: 15 minutes., cook time: 15 minutes., Total time: 30 minutes.

Ingredients:

¾ cup chopped Medjool dates.
½ cup rolled oats; ¼ cup natural peanut butter.
Chia seeds as garnish

Directions

Soak the dates in a small dish of boiling water for 5–10 minutes. Drain.

In a food processor, combine the soaked dates, oats, and peanut butter. Process until very finely chopped.

Roll into 12 balls (a scant tablespoon each). Garnish with chia seeds, if preferred. Refrigerate for a minimum of 15 minutes and up to a week.

Rice Cake Snack Sandwich

Nutrition Facts: 225 Calories, 10g fat, 31g carbs., 5g protein.

Cook Time: 5 minutes., Total time: 5 minutes., Servings: One.

Ingredients

1 tablespoon almond butter.
Two brown rice cakes.
½ teaspoon flaxseed.
A pinch of ground cinnamon.
1/2 apple, cut

Directions

Spread almond butter on one rice cake. Sprinkle with flaxseed and cinnamon. Top with the fruit and the remaining rice cake.

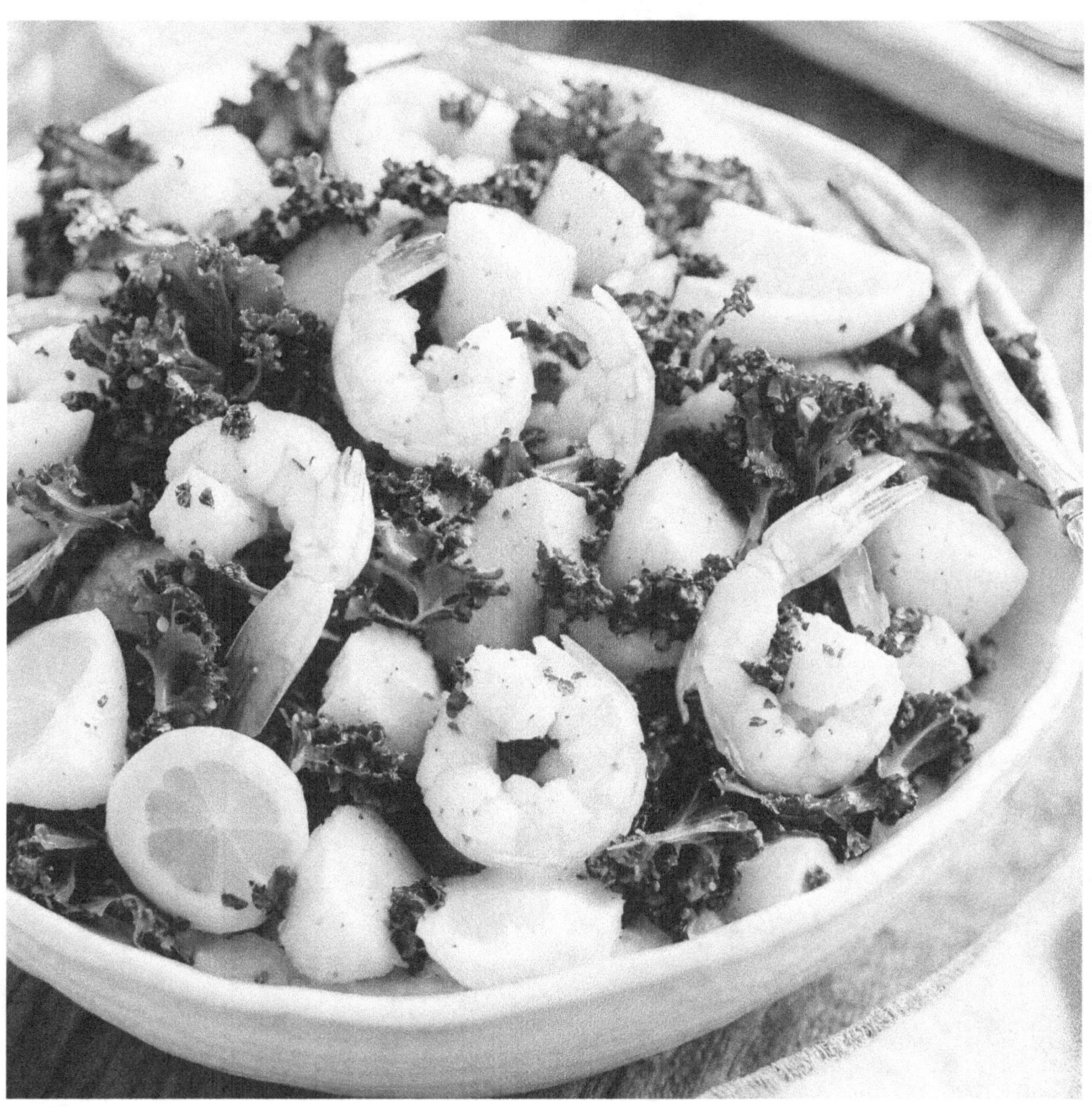

SALAD RECIPES

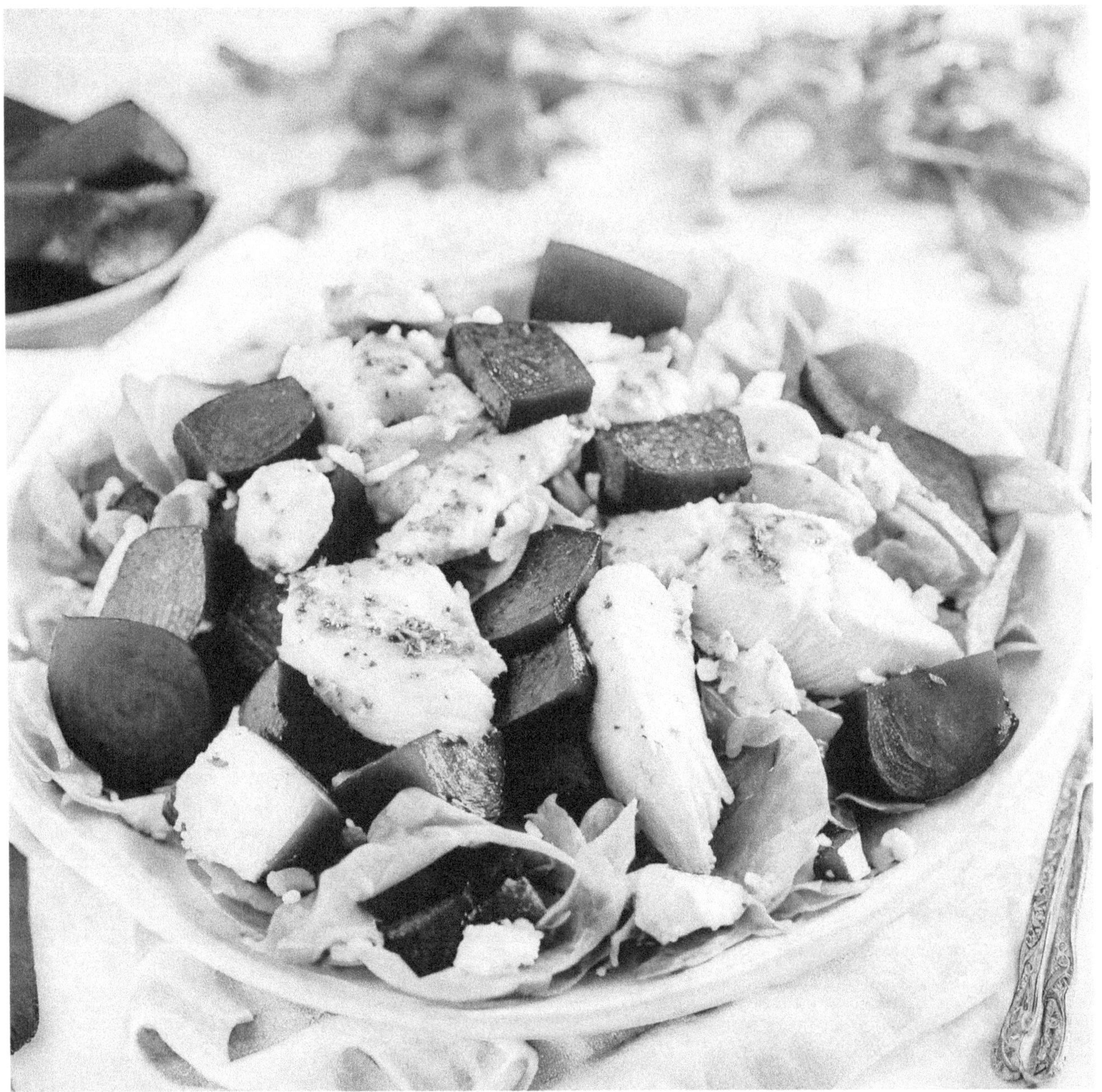

Anti-inflammatory Chicken and Beet Salad

Nutrition Facts: 380 Calories., 25g fat, 15g carbs., 24g protein.

Cook Time: 15 minutes., Total time: 15 minutes., Servings: 4

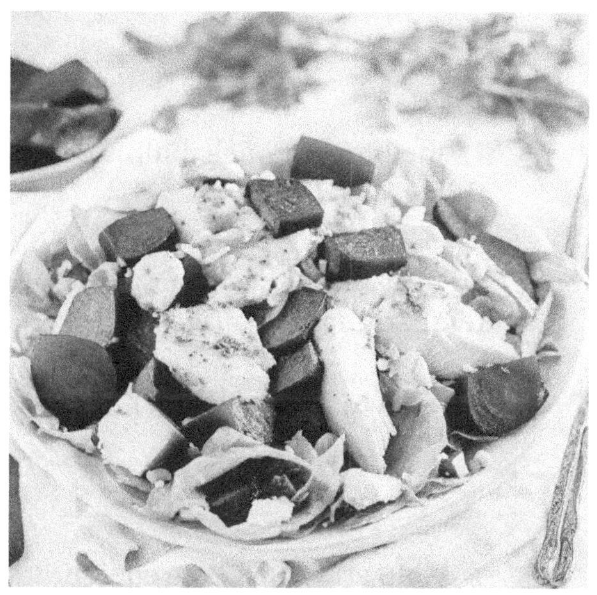

Ingredients:

- ¼ cup extra virgin olive oil.

- 2 tablespoons of tart cherry juice concentrate 1 tablespoon of white balsamic vinegar.

- 1 teaspoon salt, ¼ teaspoon powdered pepper, and ¼ teaspoon grated lime zest.

- 1 (5 ounces) package of spring mix. Salad greens

- 2 ½ cups chopped or shredded cooked chicken breast (10 oz.)

- 1 (6.7–8.8 ounces) packet of cooked beets, quartered

- ¾ cup shredded Brussels sprouts

- 1/2 cup crumbled goat cheese.

- ¼ cup chopped walnuts, toasted

Directions

In a large bowl, whisk together the oil, juice concentrate, vinegar, salt, pepper, and lime zest.

Toss together the salad leaves, chicken, beets, and Brussels sprouts. Divide the salad among four dishes and top with goat cheese and walnuts.

Kale, Quinoa, and Apple Salad.

Nutrition Facts: 499 Calories, 27g fat, 54g carbs., 13g protein.

Cook Time: 15 minutes., Total time: 15 minutes., Servings: 4

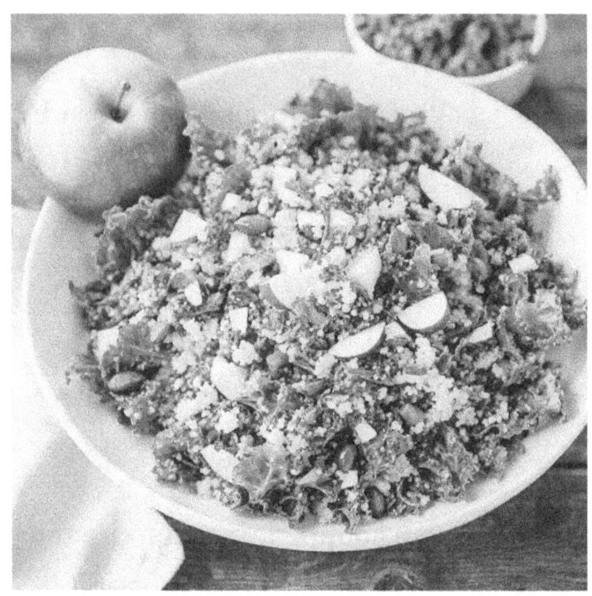

Ingredients:

- 2 teaspoons cider vinegar.

- 1 tablespoon of pure maple syrup. ½ teaspoon salt, ¼ teaspoon ground pepper, and ¼ cup extra virgin olive oil.

- 1 huge bunch of curly kale, stemmed and finely sliced (about 8 cups)

- 2 medium Honeycrisp or Gala apples, unpeeled and coarsely chopped

- 1 medium fennel bulb, cored, thinly sliced (3 cups)

- 2 cups cooked quinoa, room temperature or refrigerated.

- 1/2 cup roasted slivered almonds

- ⅓ cups dried cherries

- 1/4 cup crumbled blue cheese.

Directions

Combine vinegar, maple syrup, salt, and pepper in a large basin.

Slowly pour in the oil, stirring to mix. With clean hands, massage the kale into the dressing until it is fully coated and somewhat soft, which should take about 3 to 5 minutes.

Toss in the apples, fennel, and quinoa until evenly incorporated. Divide among four dishes, then top with almonds, cherries, and blue cheese.

Lemony Shrimp, Kale, and Potato Salad

Nutrition Facts: 522 Calories., 37g fat, 21g carbs., 28g protein

Servings: 4

Ingredients

- 3 big lemons, 1/2 cup extra virgin olive oil.

- 1 bay leaf with stem removed.

- 1 big clove of garlic, peeled 1 teaspoon honey.

- ½ teaspoon each of kosher salt and ground pepper.

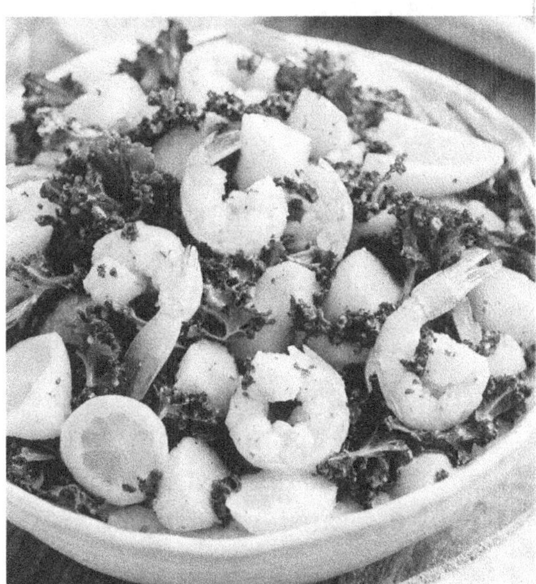

- 1 medium russet potato, peeled and cut into 1/4-inch pieces.

- 1 pound of raw shrimp (21–15 counts), peeled and deveined.

- 4 cups finely chopped stem curly kale.

- 1 pint of big cherry tomatoes, halved

- Prepare by slicing 3 small Persian cucumbers and 1/2 cup thinly sliced red onion.

- ⅓ cup pitted Kalamata olives.

- 1/2 cup crumbled feta cheese.

Directions

Cut one lemon into eight wedges and keep them aside. Cut the skin and pith from the remaining two lemons.

Working over a measuring cup, cut between the membranes and flesh to release the segments, which will fall into the cup.

Press the segments; if you don't have enough juice and fruit, squeeze one or more of the saved wedges to make up the difference.

Move the segments and liquid to a blender. Combine the oil, bay leaf, garlic, honey, pepper, and salt; blend until very smooth.

Bring 1 inch of water to a boil in a medium saucepan with a steamer basket. Spray the basket with cooking spray.

Add the potato slices, cover, and steam for 8 minutes, or until cooked. Remove from heat, then add the shrimp.

Cover and cook the shrimp in the residual heat for about 1 minute, until they become pink.

In a large bowl, toss the greens with the dressing. Massage the greens until the volume has been decreased by half. Toss in tomatoes, cucumbers, onions, and olives until well coated. Top with shrimp, potatoes, and feta. Serve with lemon wedges.

Tuna Macaroni Salad.

Nutrition Facts: 290 Calories., 11g fat, 33g carbs., 16g protein.

Cook Time: 20 minutes., Total time: 20 minutes., Servings: 6.

Ingredients:

8 ounces of whole wheat elbow macaroni.
2 (6.7-ounce) jars of tuna filets packed in water, drained
1 cup chopped celery.
1 cup of diced red bell pepper.
1/2 cup thinly sliced scallions, with more for garnish.
1/2 cup plain whole-milk Greek yogurt.
1/3 cup mayonnaise
¼ cup chopped fresh dill.
3 tablespoons of lemon juice.
1 tablespoon Dijon mustard.
½ teaspoon salt.
1/2 teaspoon of ground pepper

Directions
Cook the pasta according to the package guidelines, omitting salt. After thorough emptying, rinse with cold water until chilled. Transfer to a big bowl.

In a medium dish, shred the tuna into medium-sized bits. Stir the celery, bell pepper, scallions, yogurt, mayonnaise, dill, lemon juice, mustard, salt, and pepper into the spaghetti until thoroughly incorporated.

Gently fold in the tuna until just combined, leaving some pieces intact and taking care not to overmix. Garnish with more scallions, if desired.

Cauliflower, Quinoa, and Arugula Salad.

Nutrition Facts: 354 Calories, 25g fat, 29g carbohydrates., 9g protein.

Cook Time: 20 minutes., Total time: 35 minutes., Servings: 4

Ingredients

1 cup of water.

½ cup quinoa

6 cups cauliflower florets (1- to 2-inch chunks; from one large head, approximately 1 1/4 lbs. total)

Five tablespoons of olive oil, divided

Divide 4 tablespoons lemon juice, ¼ teaspoon salt (plus 1/8 tsp), and ¼ teaspoon ground pepper.

1 clove garlic, minced

1 tablespoon Dijon mustard.

4 cups baby arugula.

1 cup shredded carrots

1 cup grape tomatoes, halved

2 tablespoons chopped fresh dill or 2 teaspoons dried dill, and ¼ cup toasted sliced almonds.

Directions

Preheat the oven to 425°F. Quinoa and water should be combined in a small pot. Bring to a boil.

Reduce the heat to low, cover, and cook for 15 to 20 minutes, or until the quinoa is cooked and the majority of the liquid is absorbed. Fluff with a fork.

To prepare, combine cauliflower with 1 Tbsp. oil, 1 Tbsp. lemon juice, ¼ tsp. salt, and ⅛ tsp. pepper on a baking sheet.

Roast for 14 to 17 minutes, tossing once halfway through, until the cauliflower is soft and lightly browned in places. Give it five minutes to cool.

On a cutting board, use a chef's knife to create a paste by combining garlic and the remaining ⅛ tsp. salt. Transfer to a big bowl.

Combine the mustard, the remaining 3 tablespoons of lemon juice, and the remaining 1/8 teaspoon of pepper.

Whisk in the remaining 3 tablespoons of oil.Toss with the cooked quinoa, roasted cauliflower, carrots, tomatoes, and dill.

Toss gently until combined. Sprinkle with almonds.

Strawberry Spinach Salad with Avocado and Walnuts.

Nutrition Facts: 296 Calories., 18g fat, 27g carbs., 8g protein.

Prep Time: 5 minutes., Total time: 5 minutes., Servings: One.

Ingredients

3 cups baby spinach.
1 tablespoon of finely sliced red onion.
1/2 cup sliced strawberries.
2 teaspoons of vinaigrette, such as Annie's Light Raspberry Vinaigrette.
¼ medium avocado, diced
2 tablespoons of toasted walnut bits.

Directions

In a medium bowl, combine spinach, onion, and strawberries. Drizzle with vinaigrette and toss to coat. Top with avocado and walnuts.

Citrus-Lime Tofu Salad

Nutrition Facts: 390 Calories, 27g fat, 20g carbs., 25g protein.

Prep Time: 5 minutes., Total time: 5 minutes., Servings: One.

Ingredients

2 cups mixed greens.
1 cup roasted veggies, chopped if preferred

1 cup of roasted tofu
One tablespoon of pumpkin seeds.
Two tablespoons. Citrus-Lime Vinaigrette.

Directions

Place the greens, vegetables, tofu, and pumpkin seeds in a 4-cup sealable container or dish. Drizzle vinaigrette over the salad right before serving.

Quinoa, Avocado, and Chickpea Salad over Mixed Greens.

Nutrition Facts: 501 Calories, 32g fat, 47g carbs., 12g protein

Prep Time: 20 minutes., Total time: 25 minutes., Servings: Two.

Ingredients

⅔ cup water

⅓ cup quinoa, ¼ teaspoon kosher salt (or other coarse salt).

1 clove of garlic, smashed and peeled

2 tablespoons of grated lemon zest.

3 tablespoons of lemon juice.

3 tablespoons of olive oil.

1/4 teaspoon of ground pepper

1 cup of washed, salt-free canned chickpeas

One medium carrot, shredded (1/2 cup)

½ avocado, diced

1 (5-ounce) bag of prewashed mixed greens, such as spring mix or baby kale-spinach blend (8 cups packed).

Directions

Boil water in a small pot. Stir in the quinoa. Reduce the heat to low, cover, and cook for approximately 15 minutes, or until all of the liquid has been absorbed.

Use a fork to fluff and separate the grains; allow to cool for 5 minutes.

Meanwhile, sprinkle salt over the garlic on a chopping board. Mash the garlic with the side of a spoon until it forms a paste.

Scrape into a medium bowl. Whisk in the lemon zest, juice, oil, and pepper. Transfer 3 tablespoons of the dressing to a small dish and set aside.

Toss the chickpeas, carrots, and avocado with the remaining dressing. Allow 5 minutes for the flavors to mingle. Make sure to gently toss after adding the quinoa.

Toss the greens in a big dish with the leftover 3 tablespoons of dressing. Divide the greens across two dishes, then top with the quinoa mixture.

Kale and Strawberry Salad.

Nutrition Facts: 301 Calories, 28g fat, 9g carbs, 6g protein.

Cook Time: 15 minutes., Total time: 15 minutes., Servings: 4

Ingredients:

8 cups chopped lacinato kale.
Divide 5 tablespoons of extra virgin olive oil and ½ teaspoon of salt.
1 tablespoon of cider vinegar.
1 teaspoon Dijon mustard.
1/4 teaspoon of ground pepper
1 ½ cup hulled and halved fresh strawberries.
2 ounces of crumbled goat cheese with garlic and herbs
⅓ cup chopped roasted walnuts.

Directions

In a large dish, combine the kale, 2 tablespoons of oil, and 1/4 teaspoon salt.

Massage the kale with your hands for about 1 minute to ensure it is fully coated.

In a small bowl, whisk together the vinegar, mustard, pepper, and the remaining 1/4 teaspoon salt. Whisking continually, carefully sprinkle in the remaining 3 tablespoons of oil.

Add the strawberries, goat cheese, and walnuts to the kale; pour in the dressing and toss gently to incorporate.

Avocado, Tuna, and Spinach Salad.

Nutrition Facts: 432 Calories, 32g fat, 17g carbs., 20g protein.

Cook Time: 10 minutes., Total time: 10 minutes., Servings: One.

Ingredients
½ (5-ounce) can of water-packed tuna
¼ cup diced avocado
1/4 cup halved cherry tomatoes.
1 ½ teaspoons poppy seed dressing.

1 tablespoon of chopped red onion.
1 tablespoon of extra virgin olive oil.
2 cups baby spinach.
1 tablespoon of sunflower seeds.

Directions

In a medium bowl, combine tuna, avocado, tomatoes, seasoning, onion, and oil. Serve over spinach, and garnish with sunflower seeds.

Chicken, Brussels Sprouts, and Mushroom Salad

Nutrition Facts: 432 Calories, 31g fat, 15g carbohydrates., 24g protein.

Prep Time: 10 minutes., Total time: 10 minutes., Servings: 4

Ingredients:

6 tablespoons of olive oil.
3 tablespoons of red wine vinegar.
1 ½ teaspoons minced shallots
1 tablespoon Dijon mustard.
2 tablespoons chopped fresh thyme.
1/2 teaspoon of ground pepper
12 ounces of shredded cooked chicken.
4 cups shaved, fresh cremini mushrooms
4 cups of shredded Brussels sprouts
4 cups of packed baby arugula.
1 cup thinly diagonally cut celery.
1 cup shredded Parmesan cheese

Directions

In a large mixing bowl, combine the oil, vinegar, shallots, mustard, thyme, and pepper. Toss in chicken, mushrooms, Brussels sprouts, arugula, and celery. Sprinkle with Parmesan.

Grilled Caesar Salad.

Nutrition Facts: 211 Calories, 16g fat, 13g carbs., 6g protein.

Cook Time: 25 minutes., Total time: 30 minutes., Servings: 8

Ingredients:

1 big egg yolk
2 anchovy filets, coarsely minced into a paste (approximately 1 1/2 tablespoons).
½ teaspoon Dijon mustard.
½ teaspoon grated garlic.
½ teaspoon Worcestershire sauce.
¼ teaspoon salt
2 ounces grated Parmesan cheese (about 1 1/4 cups), ⅓ cup mild olive oil, and 2 teaspoons.
Two heads of romaine lettuce, outer leaves removed, were divided lengthwise through the root.
One medium lemon, halved crosswise
Four (1-inch-thick) slices of whole-grain bread

Directions

In a medium mixing bowl, combine the egg yolk, anchovies, mustard, garlic, Worcestershire sauce, salt, and 1/4 cup Parmesan.

Whisking continually, gradually add 1/3 cup oil. Cover and refrigerate until ready for use.

Preheat the gas grill on high (450°F to 500°F). Place romaine and lemon halves, cut sides up, on a large baking sheet. Drizzle with the remaining 2 tablespoons of oil and set aside.

Place the bread on unoiled grates and cook until charred and crispy, 1 to 2 minutes per side.

Move to a chopping board and put it aside. Place romaine halves and lemons, cut sides down, on unoiled grates; grill uncovered, flipping once halfway through, until the lettuce is gently charred on both sides and the lemon-cut sides are blackened, 2 to 4 minutes.

Remove from grill; set romaine on a chopping board and cut in half lengthwise (for a total of 8 wedges).

Cut the burned bread into bite-sized pieces. Mix 1 lemon half into the dressing mixture and stir until combined.

Arrange the romaine wedges on a dish; drizzle with half of the dressing mixture (about 1/4 cup), then top with the croutons.

Juice the remaining lemon half over the salad. Sprinkle with the remaining 1 cup of Parmesan. Serve immediately with the remaining dressing.

White Bean and Vegetable Salad

Nutrition Facts: 360 Calories, 25g fat, 30g carbs., 10g protein.

Prep Time: 10 minutes., Total time: 10 minutes., Servings: One.

Ingredients
2 cups mixed salad greens.
¾ cup vegetables of your choosing, such as sliced cucumbers and cherry tomatoes.
⅓ cup canned white beans, washed and strained
½ avocado, diced
1 tablespoon of red wine vinegar.
Two tablespoons of extra-virgin olive oil
¼ teaspoon kosher salt.
Add freshly ground pepper to taste.

Directions
In a medium bowl, combine the greens, vegetables, beans, and avocado. Drizzle with vinegar and oil, then season with salt and pepper. Toss to blend, then transfer to a large platter.

Cobb Salad with Herb-Rubbed Chicken

Nutrition Facts: 412 Calories., 32g fat, 11g carbs., 23g protein.

Prep Time: 35 minutes., Total time: 45 minutes., Servings: 4

Ingredients:

Chicken.
1 tablespoon of extra virgin olive oil.
1 teaspoon of garlic powder.
1 teaspoon dried thyme.
½ teaspoon dried oregano.
½ teaspoon dried rosemary.
½ teaspoon ground pepper, ¼ teaspoon kosher salt.
2 (8-ounce) boneless, skinless chicken

breasts, trimmed

Vinaigrette
⅓ cup extra virgin olive oil.
¼ cup lemon juice
2 tablespoons of champagne vinegar.
1/2 teaspoon kosher salt.
1/4 teaspoon of ground pepper

Salad
Six cups of baby kale
2 medium ripe avocados, 2 big hard-boiled eggs, 2 slices of cooked bacon (crumbled), and 1/2 cup crumbled feta cheese.
10 strawberries quartered

Directions
Preheat the grill to medium-high.
To prepare the chicken: In a small bowl, combine 1 tablespoon oil, garlic powder, thyme, oregano, rosemary, half a teaspoon pepper, and 1/4 teaspoon salt.

Rub the mixture over the chicken.

Oil the grill rack. Grill the chicken for 5 to 6 minutes per side, or until an instant-read thermometer put into the thickest section reads 160 degrees Fahrenheit.

Place the chicken on a clean chopping board and let it rest for 10 minutes. Slice.

To make vinaigrette: In a small bowl, whisk together the oil, lemon juice, vinegar, salt, and pepper.

To assemble the salad, arrange the greens, avocados, eggs, bacon, feta, strawberries, and chicken in a big dish. Serve with vinaigrette.

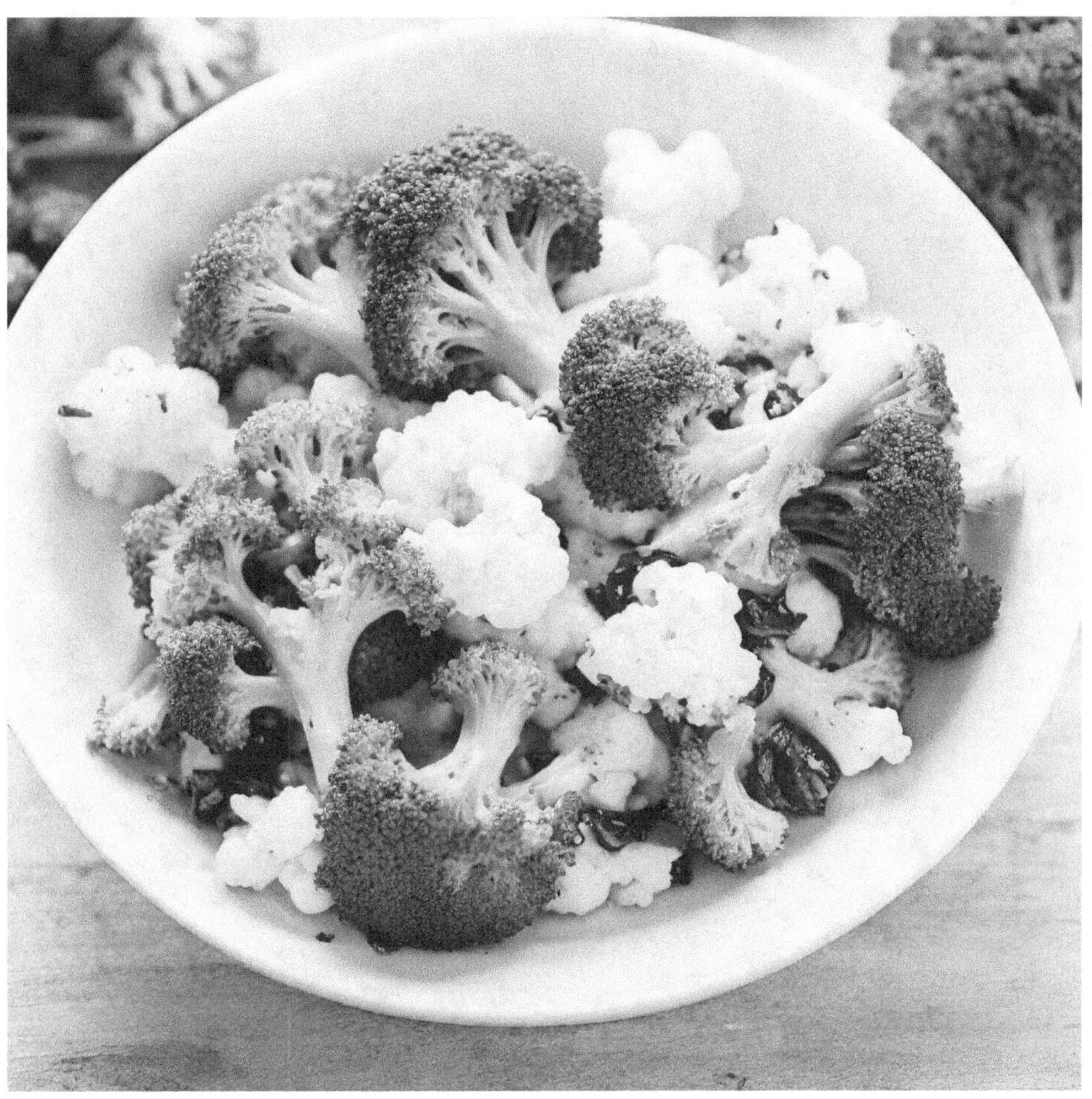

SIDE DISH RECIPES

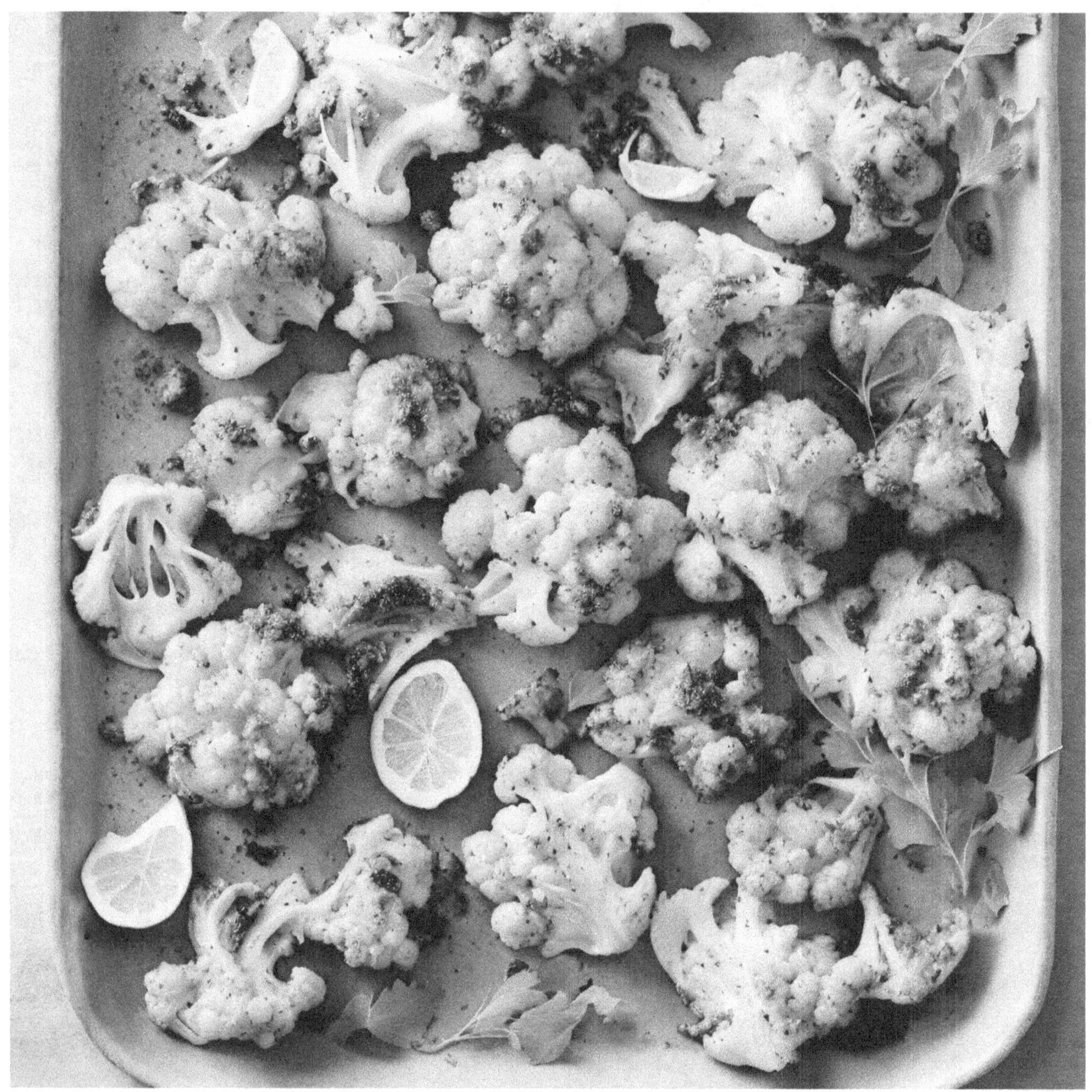

Turmeric-Roasted Cauliflower

Nutrition Facts: 124 Calories., 9g fat, 10g carbohydrates., 4g protein.

prep time: 10 minutes, Cook time: 20 minutes, Total time: 30 minutes., Servings : 5

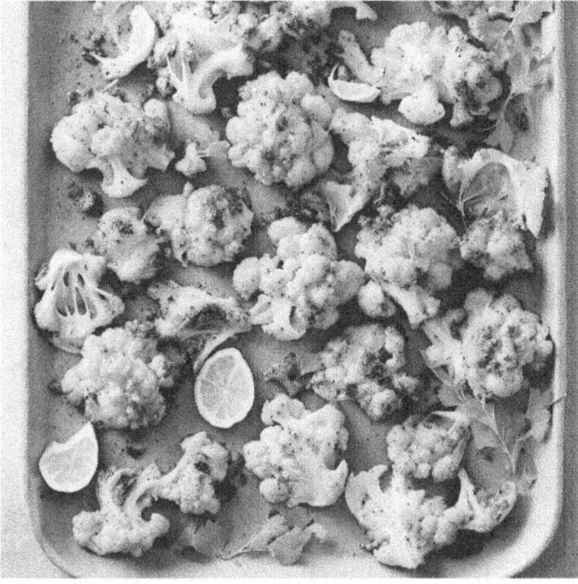

Ingredients

Three tablespoons of extra-virgin olive oil

1 ½ teaspoon ground turmeric.

1/2 teaspoon ground cumin

½ teaspoon salt.

1/2 teaspoon of ground pepper

Two big cloves of garlic, minced

8 cups of cauliflower florets (1 large head, approximately 2 pounds)

1-2 tablespoons of lemon juice.

Directions

Preheat the oven to 425°F.

In a large bowl, combine oil, turmeric, cumin, salt, pepper, and garlic. Add the cauliflower and toss to coat. Transfer to a large, rimmed baking sheet. Roast for 15 to 25 minutes, tossing once, until browned and soft. Drizzle lemon juice on the cauliflower.

Roasted Broccoli with Honey and Chipotles

Nutrition Facts: 104 Calories., 7g fat, 9g carbs., 3g protein.

Prep Time: 15 minutes., Cook time: 15 minutes, Total time: 30 minutes., Servings: 6.

Ingredients

Three tablespoons of extra-virgin olive oil

4 tablespoons honey, 1 tablespoon lemon or lime juice.

2 teaspoons of minced canned chipotles in adobo.

1 teaspoon of garlic powder.

¼ teaspoon salt

8 cups broccoli florets (about one pound)

Directions

Preheat the oven to 425 degrees Fahrenheit. Coat a large, rimmed baking sheet with cooking spray.

Combine oil, honey, juice, chipotle, garlic powder, and salt in a large mixing basin. Add the broccoli and toss to coat. Roast, tossing once, until soft and browned in places, 12 to 15 minutes.

Quinoa with Peas and Lemon.

Nutrition Facts: 148 Calories., 5g fat, 21g carbs., 6g protein.

Cook Time: 10 minutes., Total time: 10 minutes., Servings: 6.

Ingredients

1 tablespoon of extra virgin olive oil.
1 chopped onion and 1 (10-ounce) container of frozen peas.
2 cups of cooked quinoa.
Zest from 1 lemon
1/4 cup crumbled goat cheese.
¾ teaspoon salt.
1/2 teaspoon of ground pepper

Directions

In a large skillet, heat the oil over medium-high heat. Stir in the shallot and simmer for approximately 2 minutes, or until softened.

Stir in the peas and quinoa; simmer, stirring often, until cooked through, approximately 5 minutes. Stir in the lemon zest, goat cheese, salt, and pepper.

Crispy Smashed Broccoli with Balsamic and Parmesan.

Nutrition Facts: 79 Calories., 6g fat, 5g carbs., 3g protein.

Cook Time: 25 minutes., Total time: 25 minutes., Servings: 6.

Ingredients
8 cups bite-sized broccoli florets (approx. 1 pound)
2 tablespoons extra virgin olive oil,

¼ teaspoon salt, and ¼ teaspoon ground pepper.
¼ cup grated Parmesan
1 tablespoon of balsamic glaze (see Tip)

Directions
Position the oven rack 6 inches from the broiler. Preheat the broiler too high.
Bring a few inches of water to a boil in a big saucepan with a steamer basket. Broccoli should be steamed for 3 minutes or until barely tender.

Place the broccoli in an extensive baking sheet with a rim. Flatten each floret with the bottom of a Mason jar or other strong glass. Drizzle with oil, then season with salt and pepper. Evenly divide the Parmesan among the florets. Broil the broccoli for 3 to 4 minutes, or until gently browned and the cheese is melted. Drizzle with a balsamic glaze before serving.

Equipment
Large pot, steamer basket, large-rimmed baking sheet, Mason jar, or durable glass

Tip
Balsamic glaze is made by cooking balsamic vinegar until it is quite thick. Look for it with other vinegars in well-stocked shops. Alternatively, create it yourself by heating 1 cup of balsamic vinegar in a small saucepan over medium-high heat until syrupy and reduced to approximately 1/4 cup, 10 to 14 minutes.

Crispy Smashed Broccoli with Za'atar

Nutrition Facts: 70 Calories., 5g fat, 5g carbs., 3g protein.

Cook Time: 25 minutes., Total time: 25 minutes., Servings: 6.

Ingredients

8 cups bite-size broccoli florets (one pound)
2 tablespoons extra virgin olive oil
2 tablespoons za'atar

1/2 teaspoon garlic powder.
1/2 teaspoon kosher salt.
1/4 teaspoon of ground pepper
1/4 cup low-fat plain Greek yogurt

Directions

Position the oven rack 6 inches from the broiler.
Bring a few inches of water to a boil in a big saucepan with a steamer basket. Steam broccoli for 3 to 4 minutes, or until it is just tender.

Preheat the broiler too high. Spread the broccoli on a big, rimmed baking sheet.

Drizzle with oil and toss until coated. Using the bottom of a heavy glass or a mason jar, evenly distribute the florets on the pan and press them down.

In a small bowl, combine the za'atar, garlic powder, salt, and pepper. Sprinkle over the florets. Broil until heated and beginning to brown, 4 to 5 minutes.

Prior to serving, top each floret with a little dollop of yogurt.

Balsamic Broccoli and Cauliflower

Nutrition Facts: 129 Calories, 7g fat, 12g carbs., 4g protein.

Cook Time: 10 minutes, Total time: 10 minutes., Servings: 4

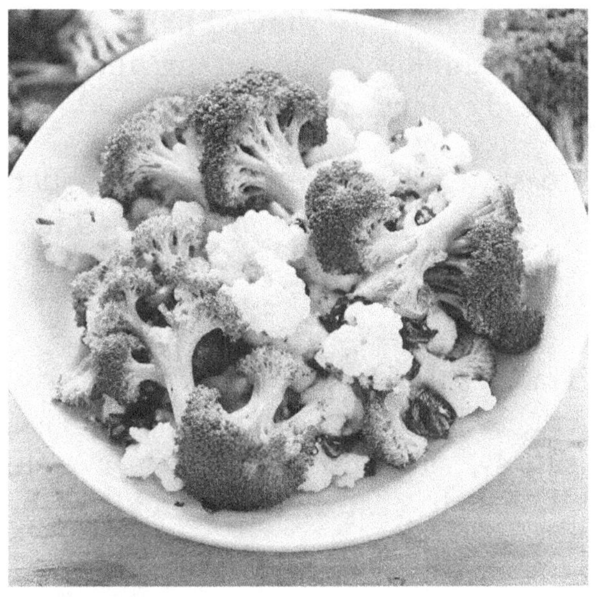

Ingredients

2 tablespoons extra virgin olive oil
Prepare by slicing 2 garlic cloves and thawing and draining a 10-ounce package of frozen broccoli and cauliflower.
2 teaspoons of balsamic vinegar.
2 tablespoons chopped fresh thyme.
½ teaspoon salt, ¼ teaspoon ground pepper.

Directions

In a large skillet, heat the oil over medium-high heat. Stir in the garlic and simmer for about a minute, or until fragrant. Stir in the broccoli and cauliflower, vinegar, thyme, salt, and pepper; simmer, stirring often, until cooked through, approximately 5 minutes.

Cauliflower "Potato Salad

Nutrition Facts: 183 Calories, 16g fat, 6g carbs., 5g protein.

Prep Time: 15 minutes., Cook time: 25 minutes, Total time: 40 minutes., Servings : 8

Ingredients

8 cups of cauliflower florets (1 1/2 to 2 inch chunks)
2 tablespoons extra virgin olive oil
1/2 cup finely sliced scallions.
½ cup mayonnaise
3 tablespoons dill pickle relish.
2 tablespoons chopped fresh flat-leaved parsley
1 ½ teaspoons coarse Dijon mustard.
1/2 teaspoon of ground pepper
3 hard boiled eggs, finely chopped.

Directions

Preheat the oven to 450 degrees Fahrenheit. On a rimmed baking sheet, toss cauliflower and oil together and spread evenly.

Roast, tossing once, until barely tender, 10 to 12 minutes. Let it cool for fifteen minutes.

Transfer the cauliflower to a large basin. Stir in the scallions, mayonnaise, relish, parsley, mustard, and pepper until completely coated. Gently fold in the eggs.

Cheesy Roasted Cauliflower

Nutrition Facts: 136 Calories, 10g fat, 8g carbs., 6g protein.

Prep Time: 10 minutes, Cook time: 25 minutes, Total time: 35 minutes., Servings: 6.

Ingredients

8 cups cauliflower florets (one large head or two tiny)

2 tablespoons extra virgin olive oil

1 tablespoon of chopped fresh herbs, such as thyme or sage.

Add ¼ teaspoon salt and ¼ teaspoon ground pepper.

¾ cup shredded cheddar cheese.

1 tablespoon of lemon juice.

Directions

Preheat the oven to 450 degrees Fahrenheit.

In a large bowl, combine the cauliflower, oil, herbs, salt, and pepper.

Move to a big baking sheet with a rim and roast for 20 minutes, rotating halfway through. Stir, then top with cheese.

Continue roasting for another 5 minutes, or until the cauliflower is tender and the cheese has melted. Toss in lemon juice and serve.

Balsamic-Parmesan Sautéed Spinach

Nutrition Facts: 84 Calories., 6g fat, 5g carbs., 3g protein.

Prep Time: 15 minutes., Total time: 15 minutes., Servings : 5

Ingredients

2 tablespoons extra virgin olive oil

3 garlic cloves, minced

1 pound fresh spinach,

¼ teaspoon salt, and ¼ teaspoon ground pepper.

2 tablespoons of grated Parmesan cheese.

4 tsp. high-quality balsamic vinegar or glaze

Directions

In a large saucepan, warm the oil over medium heat. Stir in the garlic and simmer for 30 seconds to 1 minute, or until fragrant. Toss in the spinach, salt, and pepper until coated. Stir and cook for 3 to 5 minutes, or until just wilted. Take off the stove and mix in the Parmesan. Drizzle with vinegar (or glaze), then serve immediately.

Sautéed Broccoli with Peanut Sauce

Nutrition Facts: 154 Calories., 10g fat, 12g carbs., 6g protein.

Prep Time: 15 minutes., Total time: 15 minutes., Servings: 6.

Ingredients

Eight cups of broccoli florets, chopped into 2-inch chunks

2 tablespoons of toasted sesame oil.
1 cup chopped red bell peppers
½ cup chopped yellow onions
3 medium garlic cloves, chopped.
3 tablespoons of smooth natural peanut butter.
2 ½ teaspoons of reduced-sodium tamari.
2 teaspoons of rice vinegar.
1 tablespoon of light brown sugar.
1 teaspoon cornstarch.
1 tablespoon of roasted sesame seeds.

Directions

Bring 1 inch of water to a boil in a big saucepan with a steamer basket. Add the broccoli, cover, and simmer for 3 to 4 minutes, or until tender and crisp.

Meanwhile, warm the oil in a large pan over medium-high heat. Add the bell pepper, onion, and garlic; simmer, stirring often, until the veggies soften, about 3 minutes. Stir in the steamed broccoli and simmer for 3 minutes.

In a small mixing bowl, combine peanut butter, tamari, vinegar, sugar, and cornstarch. Whisk until smooth. Stir in the veggies. Cook, stirring, until the sauce thickens, which should take approximately one minute. Sprinkle with sesame seeds.

Broccoli, Chickpea, and Pomegranate Salad

Nutrition Facts: 162 Calories, 9g fat, 16g carbs., 6g protein.

Prep Time: 10 minutes., Cook time: 10 minutes., Total time: 20 minutes.,Servings: 6.

Ingredients:

¼ cup finely sliced red onion.
1/2 teaspoon ground cumin
⅓ cup plain whole milk yogurt
2 tablespoons tahini.
2 tablespoons extra virgin olive oil
1 tablespoon of lemon juice.
¾ teaspoon salt, divided.
1/2 teaspoon of ground pepper
4 cups of bite-sized broccoli florets (approximately 8 ounces).
1 (15-ounce) can of low-sodium chickpeas, washed
1/2 cup pomegranate seeds.

Directions

Soak the onion in a small dish of cold water for ten minutes. Drain well.

Meanwhile, roast cumin in a small dry pan over medium heat, stirring until fragrant, about 1 to 2 minutes.

Transfer to a big bowl. Whisk together the yogurt, tahini, oil, lemon juice, 1/2 teaspoon salt, and pepper until smooth.

Toss in the broccoli, chickpeas, pomegranate seeds, and onion until combined. Allow it to stand for 10 minutes. Add the remaining 1/4 teaspoon salt and stir again.

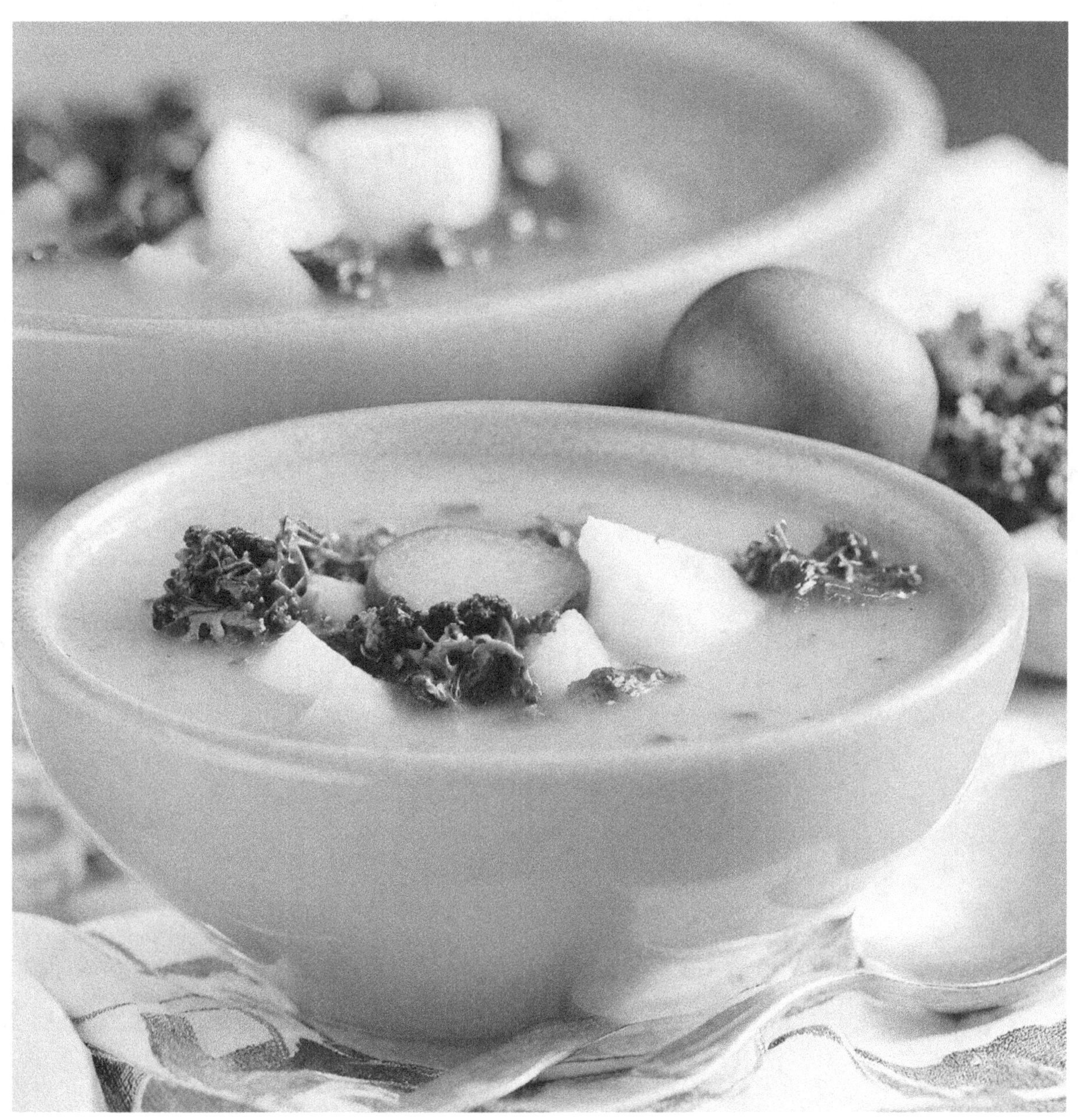

SOUP RECIPES

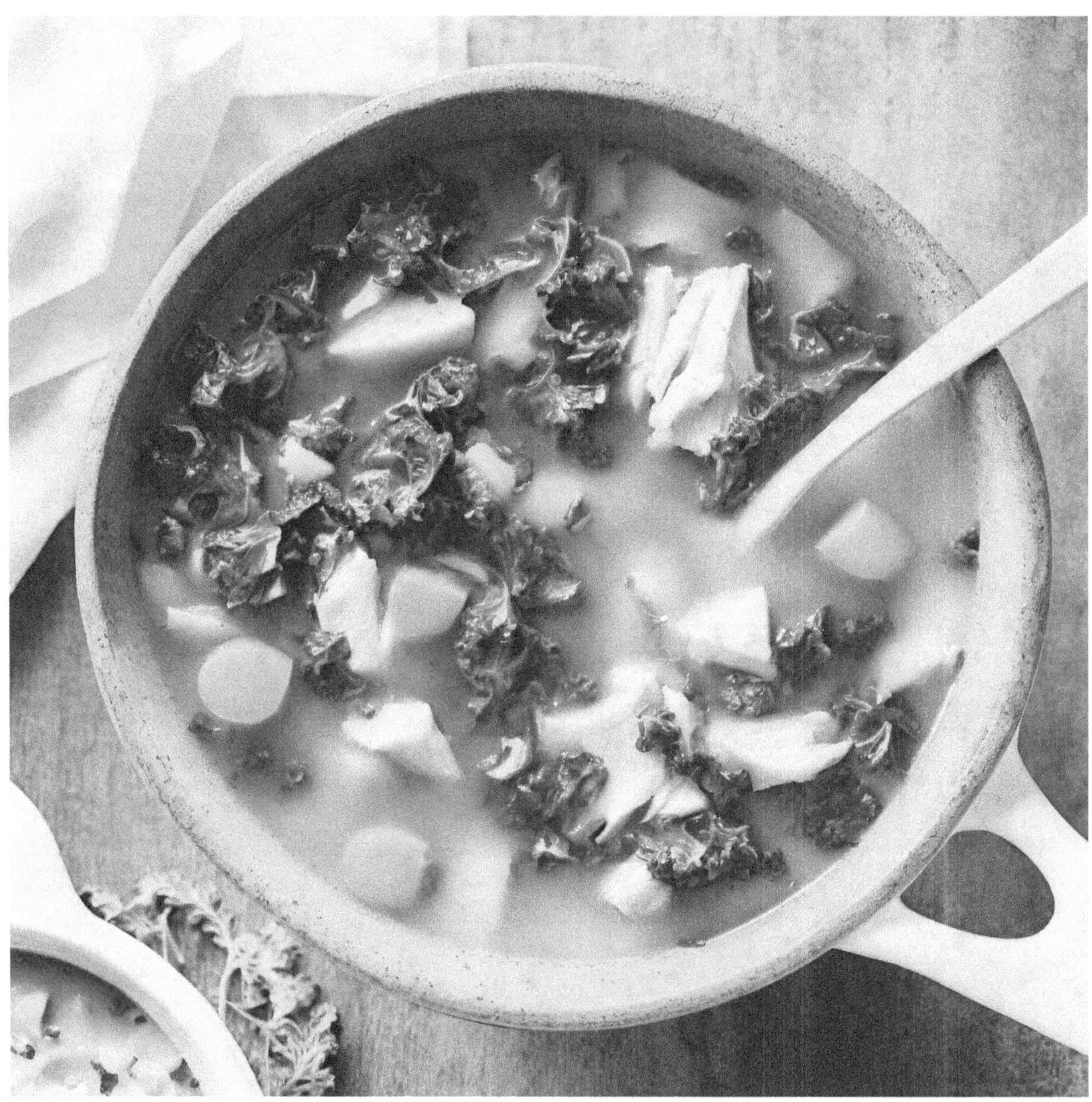

Chicken and Kale Soup.

Nutrition Facts: 271 Calories., 5g fat, 30g carbs., 26g protein.

Prep Time: 20 minutes., Cook time: 25 minutes., Total time: 45 minutes., Servings: 6.

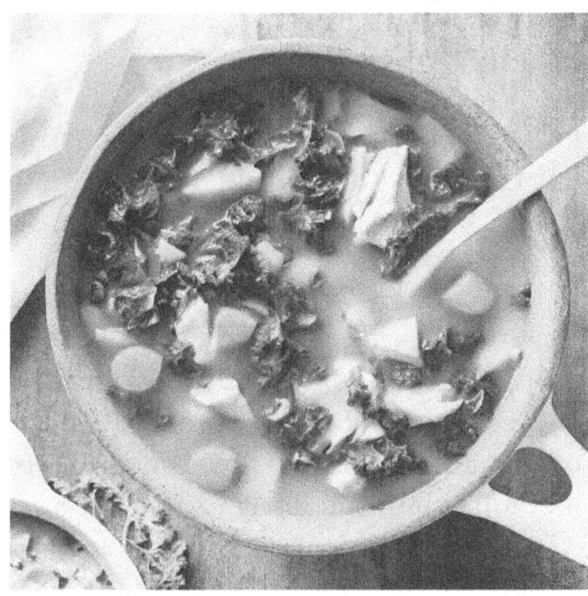

Ingredients:

1 tablespoon extra virgin olive oil.

1 ½ cups chopped yellow onion and 1 tablespoon minced garlic.

1 (15-ounce) can of no-salt-added Great Northern beans, washed

12 ounces of boneless, skinless chicken breast or chicken tenders.

Two medium Yukon Gold potatoes, peeled and diced (1/2 inch)

6 cups of unsalted chicken broth.

Three thyme sprigs

1 teaspoon of kosher salt.

1/2 teaspoon of ground pepper

3 cups chopped kale, or 1 (10-ounce) container frozen chopped kale.

2 teaspoons of lemon juice.

Directions

In a large, heavy saucepan, heat the oil over medium heat. Cook for approximately 5 minutes, stirring periodically, or until the onion is tender. Cook, stirring regularly, until the garlic is aromatic, about 1 minute. Combine the beans, chicken, potatoes, broth, thyme, salt, and pepper.

Bring to a boil over medium-high heat, then decrease heat to a simmer. Simmer, covered, for approximately 18 minutes, or until the potatoes are cooked and an instant-read thermometer inserted into the thickest part of the chicken reads 165°F.

Transfer the chicken to a platter and shred with two forks into bite-sized pieces.

Cook the kale in the broth over medium heat, stirring often, until wilted and tender, approximately 2 minutes.

Remove from the heat and mix in the shredded chicken and lemon juice. Remove the thyme sprigs before serving. Serve hot.

Creamy Sun-Dried Tomato and Spinach Soup.

Nutrition Facts: 322 Calories., 20g fat, 28g carbs., 10g protein.

Cook Time: 25 minutes., Total time: 30 minutes., Servings: 4

Ingredients

⅓ cup slivered oil-packed sun-dried tomatoes + 2 tablespoons oil from jar
2 cups of sliced mushrooms.
1 cup chopped onions
Two big cloves of garlic, minced
1 teaspoon dried basil.
1 ½ teaspoons all-purpose flour.
½ teaspoon salt.
1/2 teaspoon of ground pepper
Add 3 ½ cups of low-sodium vegetable broth and 1/2 cup of heavy cream.
4 cups of finely chopped fresh spinach.
1 (15-ounce) can unsalted cannellini beans, washed
One tablespoon of lemon juice, plus more to taste.

Directions

Heat 2 tablespoons of sun-dried tomato oil in a large saucepan over medium heat. Cook, stirring, for 3 minutes, or until the mushrooms and onion begin to soften.

Stir in the garlic and basil; simmer for 1 minute. Add the flour, pepper, and salt and stir; cook for one minute. Add the broth and cream, raise the heat to medium-high, and bring to a boil.

Reduce the heat to a simmer and cook, turning once or twice, until the veggies are tender, approximately 5 minutes.

Cook, stirring, until the spinach is wilted, approximately 2 minutes. Then, add the beans and sun-dried tomatoes. After taking off the heat, stir in the lemon juice.

Vegetarian Potato and Kale Soup

Nutrition Facts: 273 Calories., 12g fat, 38g carbs., 7g protein.

Cook Time: 45 minutes., Total time: 45 minutes., Servings: 4

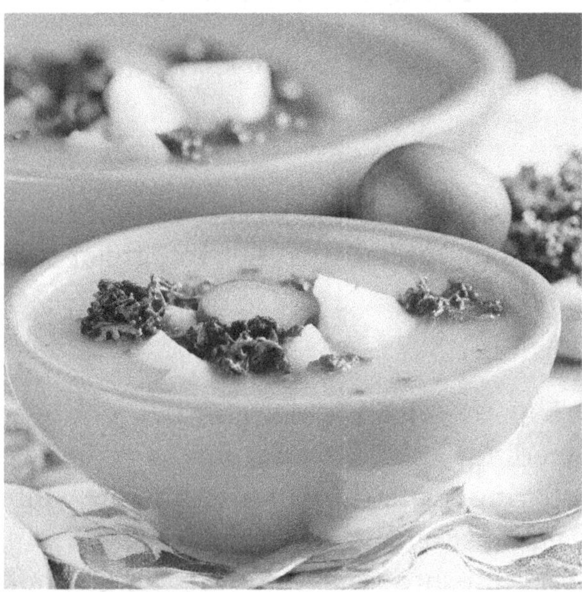

Ingredients

1 tablespoon of extra virgin olive oil.

One small, sweet onion, halved and thinly sliced

3 garlic cloves, finely chopped

4 cups low-sodium vegetable broth.

2 glasses of water.

1 pound baby red potatoes, halved lengthwise.

Two medium parsnips, peeled and sliced 1/4 inch thick.

1 teaspoon of chopped fresh rosemary, with more for garnish.

¼ teaspoon salt

1 small bunch of lacinato kale, stems, and chopped

1/2 cup grated Parmesan cheese, with more for garnish.

1/4 cup heavy cream.

1 tablespoon of lemon juice.

Directions

Heat the oil in a Dutch oven or big, heavy saucepan over medium-high heat. Add the onion and simmer, stirring occasionally, until soft, approximately 5 minutes.

Cook, stirring regularly, for approximately 30 seconds, or until the garlic is aromatic. Add the broth, water, potatoes, parsnips, rosemary, and salt; bring to a boil.

Reduce the heat to medium-low, cover, and simmer, stirring occasionally, until the veggies are soft, approximately 15 minutes. Using the back of a spoon, gently mash the veggies to thicken the soup.

Cook, stirring occasionally, until the kale is wilted, approximately 10 minutes. Add lemon juice immediately before serving. If preferred, garnish with extra rosemary and Parmesan cheese.

Shrimp and Vegetable Soup with Garlic and Ginger.

Nutrition Facts: 136 Calories, 4g fat, 10g carbohydrates., 16g protein.

Prep Time: 5 minutes., cook time: 40 minutes., Total time: 45 minutes., Servings: 6.

Ingredients:

12 ounces of fresh or frozen big shrimp, peeled and deveined; 4 green onions.
2 teaspoons of canola oil.
Two medium carrots, peeled and thinly sliced
8 ounces of fresh shiitake or oyster mushrooms, stems, and finely chopped.
1 teaspoon of powdered ginger or 1 tablespoon of freshly grated ginger.
2 garlic cloves, minced
2 (14-ounce) cans of reduced-sodium chicken broth
2 glasses of water.
1 cup edamame (shelled sweet soybeans)
1 tablespoon of reduced-sodium soy sauce.
¼ teaspoon of crushed red pepper (optional)
1 cup trimmed sugar snap peas, or roughly shredded bok choy
Slivered green onions.

Directions

If you have frozen shrimp, thaw it. Rinse the shrimp and wipe them dry with paper towels. Set aside. Slice the green onions diagonally into 1-inch-long pieces, keeping the white sections apart from the green tips. Set the green tops aside.

Heat the oil in a big, nonstick pot over medium heat. Cook for 5 minutes, stirring regularly, while adding the white sections of the green onions, carrots, and mushrooms. Add the ginger and garlic; heat and stir for another minute.

To the mushroom combination, add chicken stock, water, soybeans, soy sauce, and crushed red pepper, if preferred. After bringing to a boil, reduce the heat. Cover and boil for 5 minutes, or until the carrots are soft.

Add shrimp, pea pods, and/or bok choy to the pot. Return to boiling and lower the heat. Simmer uncovered for 2 to 3 minutes, or until the shrimp are opaque. Stir in the green onion tops shortly before serving. Garnish with slivered green onions, if preferred.

Easy Chicken and Broccoli Soup

Nutrition Facts: 433 calories, 16g fat, 24g carbs., 44g protein.

Cook Time: 25 minutes., Total time: 35 minutes., Servings: 4

Ingredients

3 tablespoons of unsalted butter.
1 ¼ cups thinly sliced leeks (white and light green portions) To prepare, cut 3 medium carrots and 2 medium celery stalks.
4 cloves of garlic, coarsely chopped
3 tablespoons of all-purpose flour.
1/2 cup dry white wine.
4 cups of unsalted chicken broth.
1 ½ cups whole milk
1/2 teaspoon of ground pepper
¼ teaspoon salt
3 cups broccoli florets (about 8 ounces)
3 cups of shredded cooked chicken breast.
2 teaspoons of lemon juice.

Directions

In a large saucepan set over medium-high heat, melt the butter. Cook, stirring occasionally, until the leeks, carrots, and celery are cooked and transparent, about 6 to 8 minutes. Reduce the heat to medium and cook, stirring frequently, until the garlic is fragrant and the flour is toasted, approximately 1 minute. Add the wine and heat, stirring frequently, until nearly totally reduced, approximately 1 minute.

Slowly add the broth, stirring constantly. Add the milk, pepper, and salt, and bring to a simmer (do not boil) over medium-high heat, stirring often and scraping the bottom of the pot to dislodge any brown pieces.

Reduce the heat to medium-low to keep the sauce simmering, then add the broccoli florets. Cook, turning occasionally, until the broccoli is cooked, approximately 8 minutes.

Add the chicken during the last 2 minutes of cooking. After taking off the heat, stir in the lemon juice. Serve immediately.

Creamy White Bean Soup.

Nutrition Facts: 185 Calories, 6g fat, 28g carbs., 7g protein.

Cook Time: 25 minutes., Total time: 45 minutes., Servings: 6.

Ingredients

2 tablespoons extra virgin olive oil
One medium yellow onion, chopped.
Three medium celery stalks, chopped.
1 tablespoon of minced garlic.
1 tablespoon of dry Italian seasoning.
1/2 teaspoon crushed red pepper.
Two (15-ounce) cans. Great Northern beans with no salt added, rinsed.
1 (2 oz) Parmesan cheese rind (optional)
4 cups of unsalted vegetable broth.
½ teaspoon salt.
1/2 teaspoon of ground pepper
One fresh or dried bay leaf.
1/2 teaspoon grated lemon zest.
2 tablespoons of lemon juice.
2 tablespoons of grated Parmesan cheese.
Chopped fresh flat-leaf parsley for garnish.

Directions

Heat the oil in a big saucepan over medium-high heat. Cook, stirring often, until the onion is transparent, which should take around 5 minutes.

Cook for approximately 2 minutes, stirring periodically, until the garlic, Italian spice, and crushed red pepper are fragrant.

Stir in the beans, Parmesan rind (if using), broth, salt, pepper, and bay leaf; bring to a boil over high heat.

Reduce the heat to medium-low and simmer, stirring occasionally, until the veggies are soft, approximately 20 minutes. Remove and discard the Parmesan rind (if applicable) and bay leaf.

Pour 2 cups of soup into a blender. Secure the cover of the blender and remove the centerpiece to let steam out.

Put a clean cloth over the entrance. Process for approximately 1 minute, or until smooth. Be cautious while combining heated liquids.

Alternatively, pour 2 cups of the soup into a medium bowl and puree until smooth using an immersion blender.

Pour the pureed soup back into the pot and stir until combined. Stir in the lemon zest and juice. Divide the soup into four bowls; top with Parmesan and parsley, if preferred.

Creamy Turkey and Vegetable Soup

Nutrition Facts: 322 Calories., 12g fat, 23g carbs, 30g protein.

Cook Time: 30 minutes., Total time: 45 minutes., Servings: 6.

Ingredients:

2 tablespoons of unsalted butter.
1 tablespoon of extra virgin olive oil.
1 ½ cups chopped leek (white and light green portions)
1 cup of finely sliced carrots.
1 cup finely sliced celery, plus leaves to garnish.
1 tablespoon of minced garlic.
2 teaspoons of fresh thyme leaves, with more for garnish.
3 tablespoons of all-purpose flour.
4 cups unsalted chicken or turkey broth.
2 cups whole milk.
8 ounces unpeeled Yukon Gold potato (1 big potato), chopped into half-inch chunks
½ teaspoon salt.
1/2 teaspoon ground pepper, with more for garnish.
4 cups shredded or coarsely chopped roasted turkey.
1 cup of frozen green peas.

Directions

Melt the butter and oil in a large saucepan over medium heat. Cook, stirring occasionally, until the leek, carrots, and celery are cooked, about 6 to 8 minutes. Cook for approximately a minute, stirring regularly, until the garlic and thyme are aromatic.

Cook, stirring regularly, until the veggies are completely covered in flour, which should take about a minute. Stir in the broth, milk, potatoes, salt, and pepper.

Turn up the heat to medium-high and boil, stirring occasionally, for approximately a minute or until the liquid begins to thicken significantly.

Reduce the heat to medium and cook, partially covered, stirring occasionally, until the potatoes are cooked, about 15 minutes.

Stir in the turkey and peas. Simmer for about 2 minutes, or until the peas are well warmed and brilliant green. If preferred, season each dish with celery leaves, thyme, and ground pepper.

Butternut Squash Soup with Avocado and Chickpeas.

Nutrition Facts: 402 Calories, 9g fat, 68g carbs., 16g protein.

Prep Time: 15 minutes., Total time: 15 minutes., Servings: One.

Ingredients:

One 15-ounce can Amy's Light-Sodium
Butternut Squash Soup
¾ cup canned chickpeas, washed
1 tablespoon of lime juice.
1 teaspoon of curry powder.
a pinch of salt.
2 tablespoons of chopped avocado.
1 spoonful of nonfat plain Greek yogurt

Directions

Heat the soup in a small saucepan with the chickpeas, lime juice, curry powder, and salt. To serve, top with avocado and yogurt.

Healthy Creamy Mushroom Soup

Nutrition Facts: 212 Calories, 12g fat, 19g carbs., 10g protein.

Prep Time: 20 minutes., Cook time: 10 minutes., Total time: 30 minutes., Servings: 6.

Ingredients

2 ½ pounds of cleaned and sliced fresh mixed mushrooms

2 tablespoons of olive oil.

2 tablespoons of unsalted butter.

1 ¼ teaspoon kosher salt.

½ teaspoon black pepper.

1/2 cup chopped shallots (from two medium onions)

1/2 cup chopped scallions (from two medium scallions)

3 tablespoons of all-purpose flour.

2 ½ cups of unsalted vegetable stock.

2 ½ cups whole milk.

2 tablespoons chopped fresh flat-leaved parsley

1 tablespoon of chopped fresh tarragon.

Directions

Roughly slice the mushrooms. Cook oil and butter in a big, heavy saucepan over medium-high heat until the butter melts.

Add the mushrooms, salt, and pepper; simmer for 8 to 10 minutes, turning often, until the mushrooms are well-browned and the liquid has gone.

Add the shallots and scallions, and simmer for approximately 4 minutes, stirring often, until tender. Add the flour and mix to blend. Add the stock and milk, stirring and scraping off any browned pieces from the bottom of the saucepan. Bring the mixture to a low boil and simmer, stirring periodically, until the broth thickens, about 5 minutes.

Remove from heat. Transfer half of the mixture to a countertop blender. Secure the cover on the blender and remove the centerpiece to enable steam to escape. Place a clean cloth over the opening and process until almost smooth. Return to the saucepan.

Alternatively, use an immersion blender to puree the soup until it is reasonably smooth but still has some intact mushrooms visible. Stir in the parsley and tarragon; serve hot.

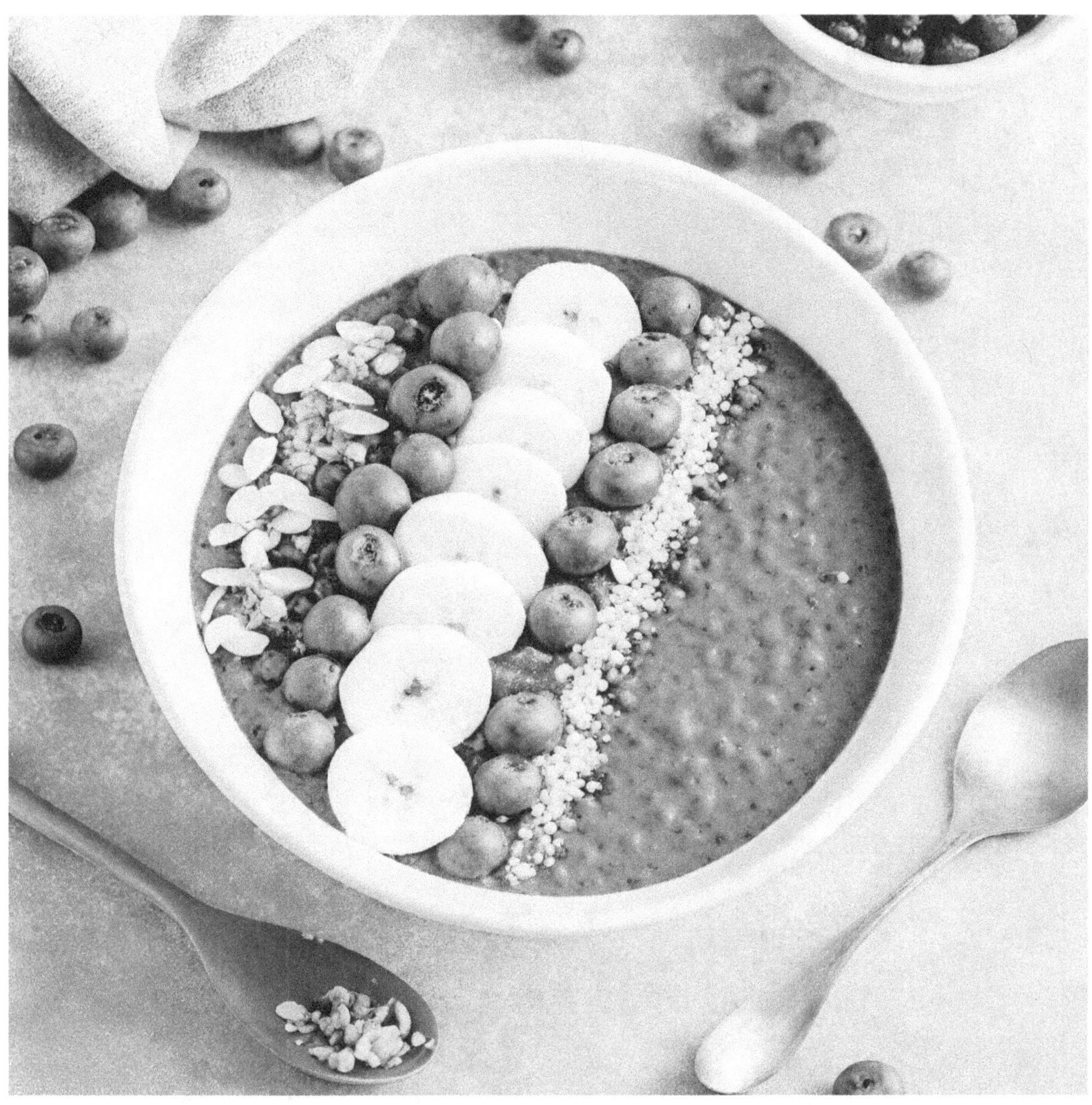

SMOOTHIE RECIPES

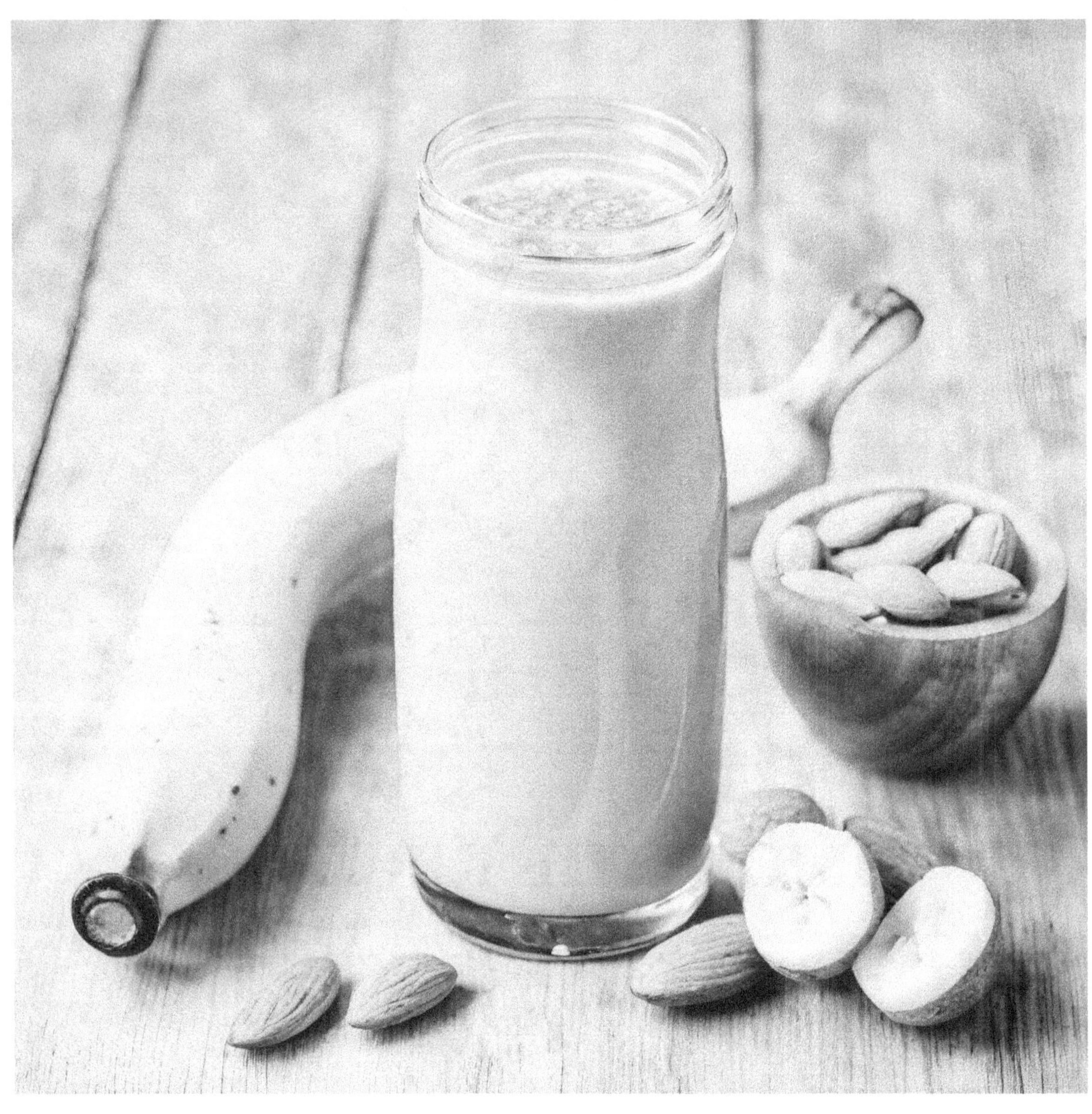

Almond Butter and Banana Protein Smoothie

Nutrition Facts: 402 Calories, 22g fat, 37g carbs, and 19g protein.

Cook time: 5 minutes., Total time: 5 minutes., Servings: One.

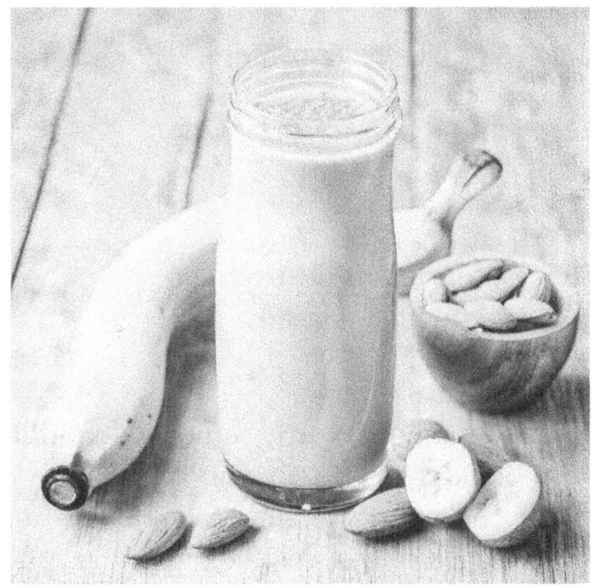

Ingredients

One tiny frozen banana.
1 cup of unsweetened almond milk.
2 tablespoons of almond butter.
2 teaspoons of unflavored protein powder.
1 tablespoon of your preferred sweetener (optional).
1/2 teaspoon ground cinnamon
4–6 ice cubes

Directions
Blend all of the ingredients until smooth.

Raspberry-Peach-Mango Smoothie Bowl

Nutrition Facts: 359 Calories, 14g fat, 46g carbs., 19g protein.

Cooking Time: 10 minutes, Total time: 10 minutes., Servings: One.

Ingredients
1 cup hulled strawberries (fresh or frozen)
½ medium banana.
1/2 cup chopped mango, fresh or frozen.

1/2 cup nonfat plain Greek yogurt
1 tablespoon of natural nut butter, such as cashew or almond.
1 tablespoon of ground flaxseed (flax meal).

¼ teaspoon vanilla extract.
Four ice cubes or one-half cup of water

Directions
In a blender, combine strawberries, banana, mango, yogurt, nut butter, flax meal, vanilla, and ice (or water). Puree till smooth.

Mango-Almond Smoothie Bowl

Nutrition Facts: 352 Calories., 9g fat, 46g carbs., 23g protein.

Cooking Time: 10 minutes, Total time: 10 minutes., Servings: One.

Ingredients
1 cup frozen mango chunks, ¾ cup nonfat plain Greek yogurt
¼ cup reduced-fat milk
1 teaspoon of vanilla essence.
¼ sliced peach
⅓ cup raspberries
1 tablespoon sliced almonds, roasted as desired
1 tablespoon unsweetened coconut flakes, toasted as desired
1 teaspoon of chia seeds.

Directions
Blend mango, yogurt, milk, and vanilla in a blender. Puree till smooth.
Pour the smoothie into a bowl and top with peach slices, raspberries, almonds, coconut, and chia seeds as desired.

Acai-Blueberry Smoothie Bowl

Nutrition Facts: 398 Calories, 14g fat, 48g carbs, 24g protein.

Cooking Time: 10 minutes, Total time: 10 minutes., Servings: One.

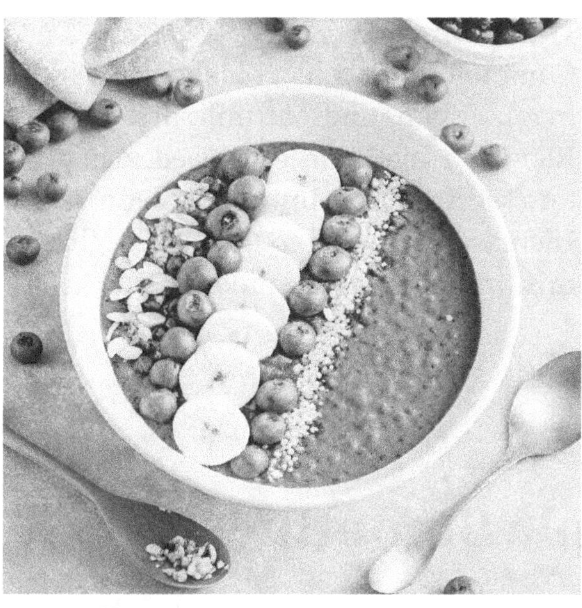

Ingredients:

¾ cup nonfat plain Greek yogurt.
3 ½ ounces of frozen, unsweetened acai fruit puree (see tip)
½ cup frozen blueberries.
½ frozen medium banana.
¼ cup coconut water
2 tablespoons of fresh raspberries.
2 tbsp. granola.
2 teaspoons toasted, unsweetened coconut flakes
1 teaspoon of chia seed.

Directions

In a blender, combine yogurt, acai powder, blueberries, banana, and coconut water. Puree till smooth. Pour the smoothie into a bowl, then top with raspberries, granola, coconut, and chia seeds.

Blueberry and Spinach Smoothie

Nutrition Facts: 342 Calories, 4g fat, 67g carbs., 11g protein.

Cook Time: 10 minutes., Total time: 10 minutes., Servings: One.

Ingredients
1 cup baby spinach.
1 cup of frozen blueberries.
1/4 cup quick or normal rolled oats.
2 teaspoons of pure maple syrup.
1 1/2 cups of oat milk

Directions
Combine spinach, blueberries, oats, maple syrup, and oat milk in a blender. Blend on medium-low speed, using the tamper if needed, until well blended. Increase the speed to medium-high, and mix until extremely smooth.

Kale and Pineapple Smoothie.

Nutrition Facts: 213 Calories, 3g fat, 41g carbohydrates., 9g protein.

Cook Time: 10 minutes., Total time: 10 minutes., Servings: One.

Ingredients
1 cup baby kale.
1/4 cup plain or coconut Greek yogurt.
1 cup of frozen pineapple pieces.
1/2 cup unsweetened vanilla coconut milk.
1/2 cup fresh orange juice.

Directions
Combine kale, yogurt, pineapple, coconut milk, and orange juice in a blender. Blend on medium-low speed, using the tamper if needed, until well blended.
Increase the speed to medium-high, and mix until extremely smooth.

Strawberry and Banana Green Smoothie

Nutrition Facts: 318 Calories., 7g fat, 48g carbs., 20g protein.

Cook time: 5 minutes., Total time: 5 minutes., Servings: One.

Ingredients
1 medium banana.
1 cup baby spinach, 1/2 cup low-fat plain
Greek yogurt.
½ cup nonfat milk.
Six frozen strawberries.
1 tablespoon flax seeds.

Directions
Blend bananas, spinach, yogurt, milk, strawberries, and flaxseeds until smooth.

Spinach, Peanut Butter, and Banana Smoothie

Nutrition Facts (Per Serving): 324 Calories., 11g fat, 45g carbs., 16g protein.

Preparation Time: 5 minutes., Total time: 5 minutes., Servings: One.

Ingredients
1 cup plain kefir.
1 tablespoon of peanut butter.
1 cup spinach.
One frozen banana.
1 tablespoon honey (optional).

Directions
Combine kefir, peanut butter, spinach, banana, and honey (if using) in a blender. Blend until smooth.

Mango Ginger Smoothie.

Nutrition Facts (Per Serving): 352 Calories., 1g fat, 79g carbs., 12g protein

Cook time: 10 minutes., Total time: 10 minutes., Servings: One.

Ingredients
½ cup cooked and cooled red lentils (see Tips).
1 cup of frozen mango chunks.
¾ cup carrot juice
1 teaspoon chopped fresh ginger
1 teaspoon honey.
A pinch of ground cardamom, plus more for garnish.
Three ice cubes.

Directions
Combine lentils, mango, carrot juice, ginger, honey, cardamom, and ice cubes in a blender. Blend on high for 2-3 minutes, or until extremely smooth. Garnish with additional cardamom, if desired.

Tips
To cook the red lentils: Cook in boiling water for approximately 15 minutes, or until just tender. Drain and chill. 2 1/2 cups cooked from 1 cup dry. Refrigerate for up to three days. Alternatively, freeze in 1/2-cup quantities for up to three months (thaw before use).

Chocolate-Banana Protein Smoothie

Nutrition facts (per serving): 310 calories., 2g fat, 64g carbs., 15g protein.

preparation time: 5 minutes., Total time: 5 minutes., Servings: One.

Ingredients
One banana, frozen
1/2 cup cooked red lentils.
½ cup nonfat milk.
2 tablespoons of unsweetened cocoa powder.
1 teaspoon of pure maple syrup.

Directions
In a blender, combine the banana, lentils, milk, chocolate, and syrup. Puree till smooth.

Pineapple Spinach Smoothie.

Nutrition facts (per serving): 151 calories., 35g carbs, 4g protein.

Cook Time: 5 minutes., Total time: 5 minutes., Servings: One.

Ingredients:

¼ cup pineapple juice.
¼ cup water
2 cups baby spinach.
1/2 cup frozen mango chunks.
1/2 cup frozen pineapple chunks.

Directions

Blend pineapple juice and water, then add spinach, mango, and pineapple. Puree until extremely smooth.

Berry-banana Cauliflower Smoothie

Nutrition Facts (Per Serving): 149 Calories., 3g fat, 29g carbohydrates., 3g protein.

Prep Time: 5 minutes., cook time: 5 minutes., Total time: 10 minutes., Servings: Two.

Ingredients

1 cup of frozen riced cauliflower.
1/2 cup frozen mixed berries.
1 cup of sliced frozen bananas
2 cups of unsweetened plain almond milk.
2 teaspoons of maple syrup.

Directions

In around three to four minutes, blend the cauliflower, berries, banana, almond milk, and maple syrup until smooth.

Pineapple Green Smoothie.

Nutrition Facts (Per Serving): 297 Calories., 6g fat, 54g carbs, 13g protein.

Cook Time: 5 minutes., Total time: 5 minutes., Servings: One.

Ingredients
1/2 cup unsweetened almond milk.
⅓ cup nonfat plain Greek yogurt
1 cup baby spinach.
1 cup frozen banana slices (about one medium banana)
1/2 cup frozen pineapple chunks.
1 tablespoon of chia seeds.
1-2 tablespoons of pure maple syrup or honey (optional).

Directions
In a blender, combine almond milk and yogurt, then add spinach, banana, pineapple, chia seeds, and sweetener (if using). Blend until smooth.

Mango-Raspberry Smoothie

Nutrition Facts (Per Serving): 188 Calories., 7g fat, 32g carbs., 2g protein.

Preparation Time: 5 minutes, Total time: 5 minutes., Servings: One.

Ingredients
½ cup water, ¼ medium avocado
1 tablespoon of lemon juice.
¾ cup frozen mango.
1/4 cup frozen raspberries.
1 tablespoon of agave (optional).

Directions
In a blender, add water, avocado, lemon juice, mango, raspberries, and agave (if desired). Blend until smooth.

Really Green Smoothie

Nutrition Facts (Per Serving): 343 Calories, 14g fat, 55g carbs., 6g protein.

Preparation Time: 5 minutes, Total time: 5 minutes., Servings: One.

Ingredients
1 big, ripe banana
1 cup packed baby kale or roughly chopped adult kale
1 cup of unsweetened vanilla almond milk.
¼ ripe avocado
1 tablespoon of chia seeds.
2 teaspoons of honey.
1 cup of ice cubes.

Directions
Blend together the banana, kale, almond milk, avocado, chia seeds, and honey. Blend on high until creamy and smooth. Add ice and mix until smooth.

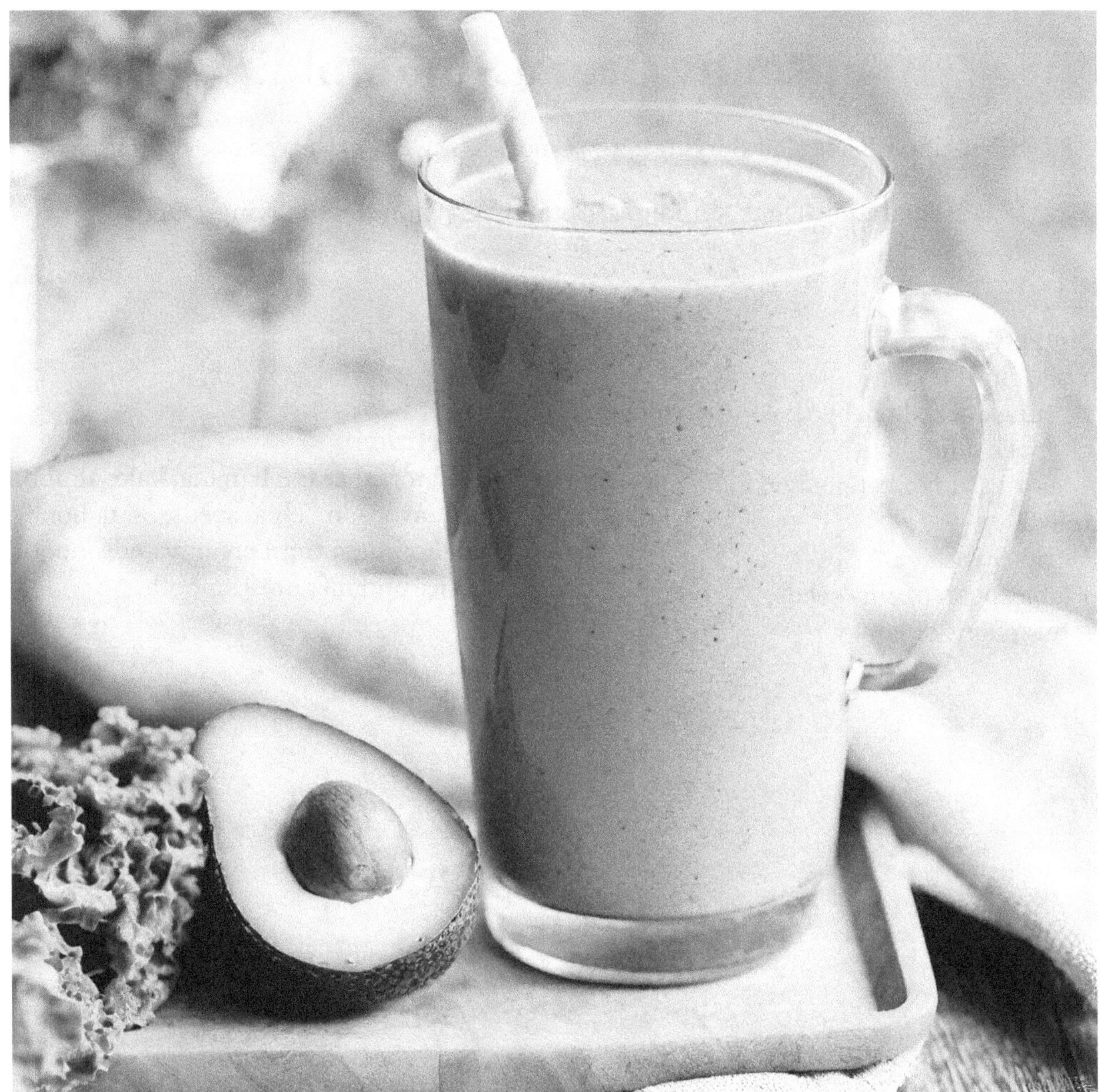

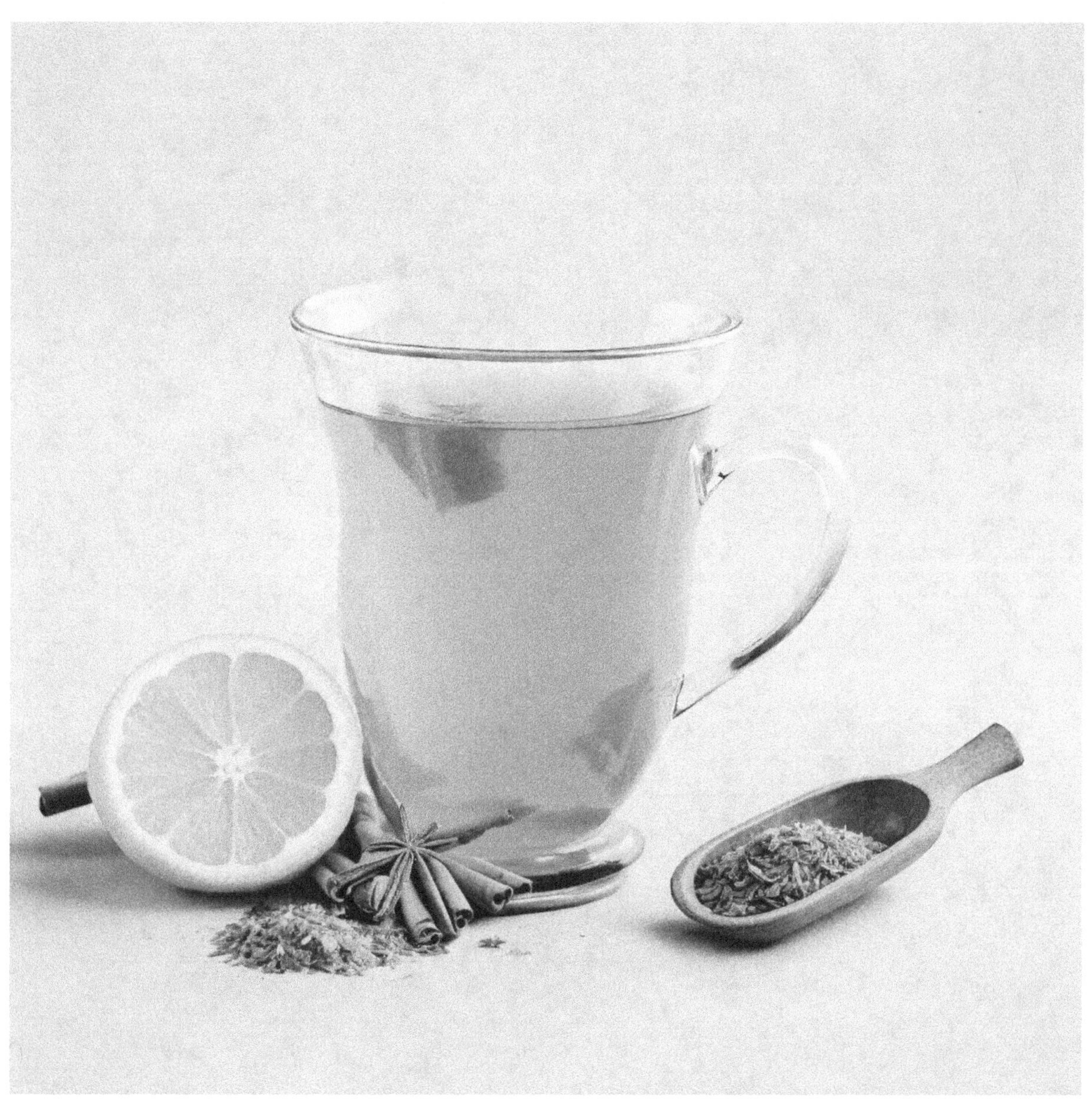

TEA RECIPES

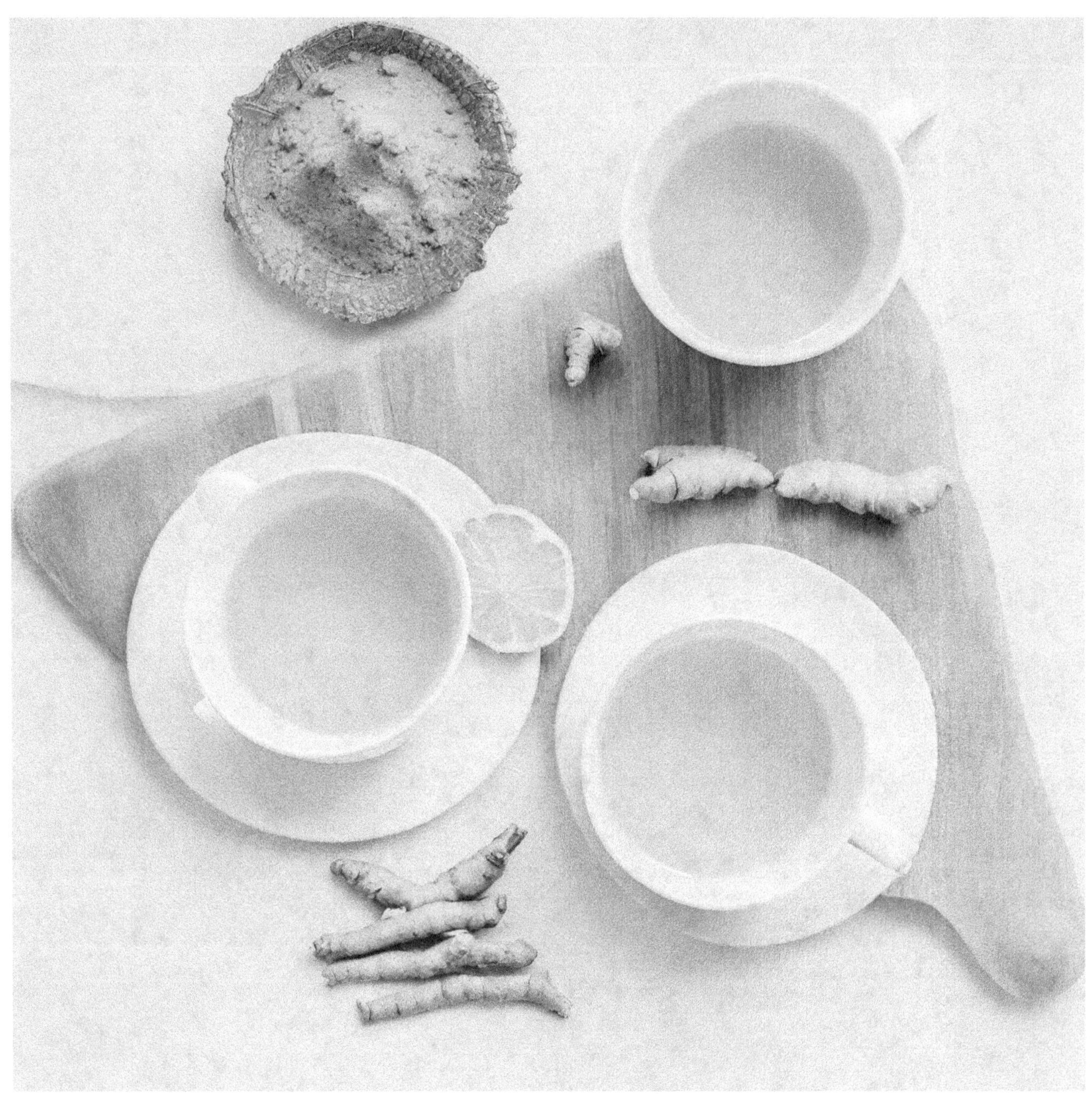

Turmeric and Ginger Tea

Prep time: 5 minutes., Serves: 2, Total time: ten minutes.

Nutritional value: low in calories, high in antioxidants and anti-inflammatory substances.

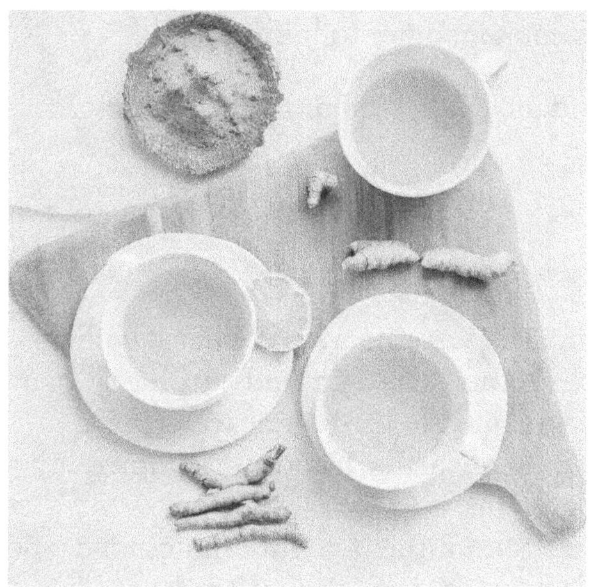

Ingredients:

2 cups water,

1 teaspoon grated fresh turmeric,

1 teaspoon grated fresh ginger,

1 tablespoon honey (optional).

Directions:

1. Heat water in a small pot till boiling.
2. Add the grated turmeric and ginger to the boiling water.
3. Reduce heat to a simmer for 5 minutes.
4. Strain the tea into mugs and add honey if desired. Enjoy it when it's hot.

Green Tea with Lemon and Mint.

Prep time: 3 minutes., Serving size: 1; total cooking time: 8 minutes

Nutritional Value: High in antioxidants, anti-inflammatory, and boosting metabolism

---

Ingredients:

one green tea bag.
Add 1 cup of boiling water and 1 lemon slice.
A few fresh mint leaves.

Directions:

1. Steep the green tea bag in boiling water for 3-5 minutes.
2. Add a lemon slice and some fresh mint leaves to the tea.

3. Allow the flavors to soak for a few minutes.
4. Remove the teabag, lemon slice, and mint leaves. Serve hot.

Cinnamon Turmeric Tea.

Prep time: 5 minutes., Servings: 2; cooking time: 10 minutes;

Nutritional value: low in calories, high in antioxidants, anti-inflammatory, and improves digestion

Ingredients:

2 cups water,

1 teaspoon ground turmeric,

1/2 teaspoon ground cinnamon.
one spoonful of honey (optional).

Directions:

1. Heat water in a small pot till boiling.
2. Add the ground turmeric and cinnamon to the boiling water.
3. Reduce the heat to a simmer for 5 minutes.
4. Strain the tea into mugs and add honey if desired. Enjoy it when it's hot.

Chamomile Lavender Tea.

Prep time: 5 minutes., Serving size: 1; preparation time: 10 minutes

Nutritional benefits: calming, anti-inflammatory, and digestive assistance

---

Ingredients:

one chamomile tea bag.
Add 1 cup of boiling water and 1 teaspoon of dried lavender.

Directions:

Step 1: Steep a chamomile tea bag and dried lavender in boiling water for 5 minutes.
2. Strain the tea into a cup. Enjoy it when it's hot.

Hibiscus Rosehip Tea

Prep time: 5 minutes., Servings: 2; total time: 10 min.
Nutritional value: high in vitamin C, antioxidants, and anti-inflammatory

---

Ingredients:

2 cups water;

2 teaspoons dried hibiscus flowers.
One spoonful of dried rosehips
Honey or Stevia (optional)

Directions:

1. Heat water in a small pot till boiling.
2. Place the rosehips and dried hibiscus blossoms into the boiling water.
3. Reduce the heat to a simmer for 5 minutes.
4. Strain the tea into mugs, then sweeten with honey or stevia if preferred. Enjoy hot or cold.

Lemon and Ginger Tea

Prep time: 5 minutes., Servings: 2; total time: 10 min.
Nutritional Value: Rich in vitamin C, antioxidants, anti-inflammatory properties, and improves digestion

---

Ingredients:

2 cups water;

1 inch of finely sliced fresh ginger;
lemon juice
Honey (optional)

Directions:

1. Heat water in a small pot till boiling.
2. Add the ginger slices to the boiling water.
3. Simmer for 5 minutes, then remove from the heat.
4. Add lemon juice and honey, if preferred. Strain into glasses, and serve hot.

Peppermint Tea

Prep time: 5 minutes., Serving size: 1; preparation time: 10 minutes

Nutritional benefits: soothing, digestive assistance, and anti-inflammatory characteristics

---

Ingredients:
one peppermint tea bag.
One cup of hot water

Directions

1. Steep the peppermint tea bag in boiling water for 5 minutes.
2. Remove the tea bag and drink it hot.

Rooibos Tea with Orange and Cinnamon

Prep time: 5 minutes., Servings: 2; Time: 10 minutes;

Nutritional value: high in antioxidants, anti-inflammatory, and caffeine-free.

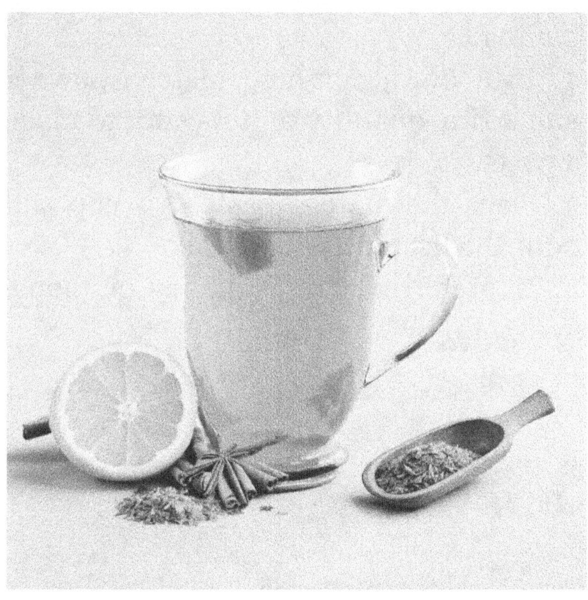

Ingredients:

2 cups of water.
two Rooibos tea bags.
one orange, sliced
one cinnamon stick.

Directions:

1. Heat water in a small pot till boiling.
2. Add rooibos tea bags, orange slices, and a cinnamon stick to the boiling water.
3. Reduce the heat to a simmer for 5 minutes.
4. Remove the teabags, orange slices, and cinnamon sticks. Serve hot.

Matcha Green Tea Lattes

Prep time: 5 minutes., Serving size: 1; preparation time: 10 minutes;

Nutritional benefits: high in antioxidants, anti-inflammatory, and metabolism -boosting

---

Ingredients:

1 teaspoon matcha green tea powder
1 cup unsweetened almond milk (or whatever milk you want)
One teaspoon of honey or maple syrup (optional)

Directions:

1. Heat almond milk in a small saucepan over medium heat until hot but not boiling.
2. In a bowl, combine matcha powder and a tiny quantity of hot water to make a paste.
3. Place the matcha paste in a cup and pour the heated almond milk.
4. If preferred, stir in honey or maple syrup. Enjoy when hot.

Berry-Hibiscus Tea

Prep time: 5 minutes., Servings: 2; total time: 10 min.
Nutritional Value: High in antioxidants, vitamin C, anti-inflammatory properties, and immunological support.

Ingredients:

2 cups of water;

2 hibiscus tea bags.
1/2 cup mixed berries (strawberries, raspberries, and blueberries).
Honey or Stevia (optional)

Directions:

1. Heat water in a small pot till boiling.
2. Combine the hibiscus tea bags and mixed berries in the boiling water.

3. Reduce the heat to a simmer for 5 minutes.
4. Remove the teabags and berries. Strain the tea into mugs, then sweeten with honey or stevia, if preferred. Enjoy hot or cold

MEAL PLANNING

Introduction to Meal Planning for an Anti-Inflammatory Diet:

Meal planning is a key component of successfully adopting an anti-inflammatory diet. By carefully selecting and preparing meals that incorporate anti-inflammatory foods while avoiding those that may contribute to inflammation, you can optimize your health and well-being. This comprehensive guide will walk you through the steps of meal planning for an anti-inflammatory diet, including tips for selecting ingredients, creating balanced meals, and staying organized.

Step 1: Understand Anti-Inflammatory Foods:

Before you start meal planning, it's essential to familiarize yourself with the types of foods that are beneficial for reducing inflammation. Anti-inflammatory foods include:

1. Fruits: Berries (such as strawberries, blueberries, and raspberries), cherries, oranges, and pineapple.

2. Vegetables: Leafy greens (like spinach, kale, and Swiss chard), cruciferous vegetables (such as broccoli, Brussels sprouts, and cauliflower), peppers, tomatoes, and sweet potatoes.

3. Whole Grains: Quinoa, brown rice, oats, barley, and whole wheat.

4. Healthy Fats: Olive oil, avocado oil, nuts (such as almonds, walnuts, and pistachios), seeds (like flaxseeds, chia seeds, and hemp seeds), and fatty fish (including salmon, mackerel, and sardines).

5. Lean Protein: Beans (such as black beans, chickpeas, and lentils), tofu, tempeh, poultry (like chicken and turkey), and eggs.

6. Herbs and Spices: Turmeric, ginger, garlic, cinnamon, and rosemary.

Step 2: Plan Your Meals:

Once you're familiar with anti-inflammatory foods, it's time to plan your meals. Follow these steps to develop a balanced meal plan:

1. Set Goals: Determine your dietary goals, such as incorporating more fruits and vegetables, reducing processed foods, or increasing omega-3 fatty acids.

2. Choose Recipes: Select recipes that feature anti-inflammatory ingredients and align with your dietary goals. Look for a variety of breakfast, lunch, dinner, and snack options to keep your meals interesting.

3. Consider Balance: Aim to include a balance of macronutrients (carbohydrates, protein, and fat) in each meal. Incorporate a variety of colorful fruits and vegetables to ensure you're getting a wide range of vitamins, minerals, and antioxidants.

4. Plan Ahead: Take time each week to plan your meals and create a grocery list. Consider batch cooking or preparing components of meals in advance to save time during the week.

5. Be Flexible: Allow for flexibility in your meal plan to accommodate changes in schedule, unexpected events, or personal preferences. It's okay to swap out recipes or ingredients as needed.

Step 3: Grocery Shopping:

Once you've planned your meals, it's time to head to the grocery store. Use these tips to make your shopping trip a success:

1. Stick to Your List: Bring your meal plan and grocery list with you to the store, and try to stick to the items you've planned to purchase.

2. Shop the Perimeter: Focus on shopping the perimeter of the store, where you'll find fresh produce, lean proteins, and whole grains. Limit your exposure to processed and packaged foods in the inner aisles.

3. Read Labels: When selecting packaged foods, read the ingredient list and nutrition label to identify any potential inflammatory ingredients, such as added sugars, trans fats, or artificial additives.

4. Buy in Bulk: Consider purchasing non-perishable items like grains, beans, nuts, and seeds in bulk to save money and reduce waste.

5. Choose Seasonal Produce: Opt for seasonal fruits and vegetables whenever possible, as they tend to be fresher, more flavorful, and more affordable.

Step 4: Meal Preparation:

Once you've returned from the grocery store, it's time to prepare your meals. Follow these tips to streamline the meal preparation process:

1. Wash and Chop Produce: Wash and chop fruits and vegetables as soon as you get home from the store to make meal prep quicker and easier throughout the week.

2. Batch Cook: Consider batch cooking grains, proteins, and vegetables in advance to have on hand for quick and convenient meals. Cook a large batch of quinoa, roast a tray of vegetables, or grill several chicken breasts to use in multiple meals throughout the week.

3. Use Time-Saving Tools: Take advantage of time-saving kitchen tools like a slow cooker, Instant Pot, or food processor to streamline meal preparation and cooking.

4. Portion Out Meals: Portion out meals into individual containers for easy grab-and-go lunches or dinners during the week. This can help prevent overeating and ensure you have balanced meals ready to go.

Step 5: Stay Organized and Flexible:

Finally, stay organized and flexible as you navigate your anti-inflammatory meal plan. Use these strategies to stay on track:

1. Keep a Meal Calendar: Use a meal planning calendar or app to track your meals for the week and stay organized.

2. Rotate Recipes: Rotate recipes regularly to keep meals interesting and prevent boredom. Experiment with new ingredients and flavors to keep your taste buds satisfied.

3. Listen to Your Body: Pay attention to how your body responds to different foods and adjust your meal plan accordingly. Everyone's dietary needs and preferences are unique, so it's important to listen to your body and make adjustments as needed.

4. Seek Support: Consider enlisting the support of family members, friends, or a registered dietitian as you embark on your anti-inflammatory meal plan journey. Having support and accountability can keep you motivated and guide you on the right track.

28 DAYS ANTI INFLAMMATORY DIET MEAL PLAN

Week 1:

Day 1:

- Breakfast: Spinach & Egg Scramble with Raspberries

- Lunch: Veggie & Hummus Sandwich

- Dinner: Chicken & Kale Taco Salad with Jalapeño-Avocado Ranch

Day 2:

- Breakfast: Avocado & Kale Omelet

- Lunch: Black Bean-Quinoa Bowl

- Dinner: Shrimp bowl over brown rice with avocado and tomatoes.

Day 3:

- Breakfast: Baby Kale Breakfast Salad with Smoked Trout & Avocado

- Lunch: Chickpea Tuna Salad

- Dinner: Baked Fish Tacos with Avocado

Day 4:

- Breakfast: Avocado & Arugula Omelet

- Lunch: Lemony Lentil Salad with Feta

- Dinner: Quinoa Chickpea Salad with Roasted Red Pepper Hummus Dressing

Day 5:

- Breakfast: Smoked Trout & Spinach Scrambled Eggs

- Lunch: Loaded Cucumber & Avocado Sandwich

- Dinner: Cauliflower Rice Bowls with Grilled Chicken

Day 6:

- Breakfast: Breakfast Beans with Microwave-Poached Egg

- Lunch: Avocado Tuna Spinach Salad

- Dinner: Sheet-Pan Chili-Lime Salmon with Potatoes & Peppers

Day 7:

- Breakfast: Avocado & Smoked Salmon Omelet

- Lunch: Vegan Burrito Bowls with Cauliflower Rice

- Dinner: Creamy Spinach Pasta

Week 2:

Day 8:

- Breakfast: Avocado-Egg Toast

- Lunch: Arugula & Cucumber Salad with Tuna

- Dinner: Lemon-Garlic Pasta with Salmon

Day 9:

- Breakfast: Smoked Salmon Scrambled Eggs

- Lunch: Mediterranean Tuna-Spinach Salad

- Dinner: Crispy Fish Taco Bowls

Day 10:

- Breakfast: Beans on Toast

- Lunch: Quinoa, Avocado & Chickpea Salad over Mixed Greens

- **Dinner: Salmon-Stuffed Avocados**

Day 11:

- **Breakfast: Feta, Egg & Olive Pita**

- **Lunch: Sweet Potato & Cauliflower Rice Bowl**

- **Dinner: Vegan Coconut Chickpea Curry**

Day 12:

- **Breakfast: Chickpea & Kale Toast**

- **Lunch: Chicken, Avocado & Quinoa Bowls with Herb Dressing**

- **Dinner: Salmon Tacos with Pineapple Salsa**

Day 13:

- **Breakfast: Berry-Orange Chia Pudding**

- **Lunch: Vegan Grain Bowl**

- **Dinner: Skillet Lemon Chicken with Spinach**

Day 14:

- **Breakfast: Rosemary, tomato, and feta egg sandwiches.**

- **Lunch: Avocado Toast with Burrata**

- **Dinner: Salmon with Lemon-Herb Orzo & Broccoli**

Week 3:

Day 15:

- **Breakfast: Skillet Eggs with Tomatillos & Spinach**

- **Lunch: Stuffed Sweet Potato with Hummus Dressing**

- **Dinner: Quinoa Chili with Sweet Potatoes**

Day 16:

- **Breakfast: Spinach & Egg Sweet Potato Toast**

- **Lunch: White Bean & Veggie Salad**

- **Dinner: Creamy Salmon Pasta with Sun-Dried Tomatoes**

Day 17:

- **Breakfast: Two-Ingredient Banana Pancakes**

- **Lunch: Quick Lentil Salmon Salad**

- **Dinner: One-Pot Chicken & Broccoli Pasta**

Day 18:

- **Breakfast: Egg Salad Avocado Toast**

- **Lunch: Roasted Veggie & Tofu Brown Rice Bowl**

- **Dinner: Kale & Quinoa Salad with Lemon Dressing**

Day 19:

- **Breakfast: Smoked Salmon & Cream Cheese Omelet**

- **Lunch: Salmon Salad-Stuffed Avocado**

- **Dinner: One-Pot Garlicky Shrimp & Spinach**

Day 20:

- **Breakfast: Spinach & Feta Scrambled Egg Pitas**

- **Lunch: Kale, Quinoa & Apple Salad**

- **Dinner: Quinoa with Chickpeas Roasted red pepper sauce**

Day 21:

- Breakfast: Avocado & Smoked Salmon Omelet

- Lunch: Chicken & Kale Taco Salad with Jalapeño-Avocado Ranch

- Dinner: Shrimp bowl over brown rice with avocado and tomatoes.

Week 4:

Day 22:

- Breakfast: Avocado & Kale Omelet

- Lunch: Veggie & Hummus Sandwich

- Dinner: Baked Fish Tacos with Avocado

Day 23:

- Breakfast: Baby Kale Breakfast Salad with Smoked Trout & Avocado

- Lunch: Chickpea Tuna Salad

- Dinner: Quinoa Chickpea Salad with Roasted Red Pepper Hummus Dressing

Day 24:

- Breakfast: Avocado & Arugula Omelet

- Lunch: Lemony Lentil Salad with Feta

- Dinner: Cauliflower Rice Bowls with Grilled Chicken

Day 25:

- Breakfast: Smoked Trout & Spinach Scrambled Eggs

- Lunch: Loaded Cucumber & Avocado Sandwich

- Dinner: Sheet-Pan Chili-Lime Salmon with Potatoes & Peppers

Day 26:

- **Breakfast: Breakfast Beans with Microwave-Poached Egg**

- **Lunch: Avocado Tuna Spinach Salad**

- **Dinner: Creamy Spinach Pasta**

Day 27:

- **Breakfast: Avocado-Egg Toast**

- **Lunch: Arugula & Cucumber Salad with Tuna**

- **Dinner: Lemon-Garlic Pasta with Salmon**

Day 28:

- **Breakfast: Smoked Salmon Scrambled Eggs**

- **Lunch: Mediterranean Tuna-Spinach Salad**

- **Dinner: Crispy Fish Taco Bowls**

CONCLUSION

"Anti-Inflammatory Diet Cookbook for Beginners" serves as a comprehensive guide to adopting a dietary approach that promotes optimal health and well-being. Throughout this book, we've explored the principles of the anti-inflammatory diet, learned about the importance of incorporating nutrient-rich, whole foods while minimizing processed and inflammatory ingredients.

By following the recipes and meal plans provided in this book, beginners can embark on a journey towards better health and vitality. From flavorful breakfast options to satisfying lunches and dinners, each recipe is carefully crafted to feature anti-inflammatory ingredients and delicious flavors. Whether you're seeking to reduce inflammation, manage chronic health conditions, or simply improve your overall health, this cookbook provides the tools and resources you need to get started on your anti-inflammatory diet journey.

As you continue your culinary exploration, remember to listen to your body, experiment with new ingredients and flavors, and enjoy the nourishing benefits of wholesome, anti-inflammatory foods. With dedication, mindfulness, and a commitment to lifelong wellness, you can harness the power of nutrition to support your health goals and thrive on your journey towards optimal well-being.

Thank you for joining us on this journey towards a healthier, more vibrant life through the anti-inflammatory diet. Here's to delicious meals, vibrant health, and a lifetime of wellness!

Anne .J. Baker

www.ingramcontent.com/pod-product-compliance
Lightning Source LLC
Chambersburg PA
CBHW080719260726
48660CB00010B/3603